EDWARD BACH
AND YOUR
EVOLUTIONARY PURPOSE

'A profound but sensitive work that unifies key ideas and practices to help us appreciate the symbiosis of spiritual, emotional and physical states – and access subtle clues to healing. The author draws together a deeper understanding of Bach's healing motivations and methods for his Twelve Healers and later-discovered remedies – including a private appreciation of connections between Moon signs and personality types – with the notion of the soul's progress, challenges and potential harmony. Alongside, she demonstrates how Evolutionary Astrology's focus on lunar Nodes elucidates further pointers towards soul purpose and karmic reconciliation. Gaye Mack's extensive, practical experience and wide range of references within Mind, Body and Spirit literature enable her to provide a sound explanation of chakra energy integration, while delivering an eloquent, in-depth appreciation of the gentle, yet significant, power of flower remedies to offer simple, easy-to-access healing opportunities – as former Harley Street doctor, Edward Bach, wholeheartedly intended.'

Diana McMahon Collis

Diana writes the Moon phases column for The Mountain Astrologer *journal and is a Mind, Body and Spirit, non-fiction editor with Oxford-based Jericho Writers*

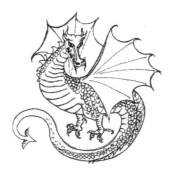

Edward Bach
and your
Evolutionary
Purpose

Gaye Mack

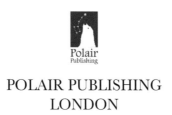

POLAIR PUBLISHING
LONDON

A fully revised and augmented edition of
IGNITING SOUL FIRE, first published 2004
EDWARD BACH AND YOUR EVOLUTIONARY PURPOSE is
First published 2021

British Library Cataloguing-in-Publication Data
A catalogue reference for this book is available
from the British Library

ISBN 978-1-905398-54-6

The author is appreciative of the White Eagle Lodge in granting
permission to make a series of quotations from publications of the
White Eagle Publishing Trust, which are ©The White Eagle
Lodge–Publishing. She also appreciates the generosity of Julian
Barnard, Steven Forrest and Carolyn Myss in allowing their
copyrighted work to be quoted in both this
volume and the one it replaces.

Printed in Great Britain by the
Halstan Printing Printing Group
Amersham

CONTENTS

ONE

—

You Have a Plan and the Universe Laughs

THE UNIVERSE was certainly laughing in the mid-1980s when I was entrenched in what I thought was the 'dream' corporate job of my life. Suddenly my health took a serious dive. As a result, I entered a period of several years during which I had a lot of tests and was examined by many specialists. While each was well qualified in their field, none seemed to have the definitive answer and my health continued to deteriorate. Finally, a friend suggested I seek an evaluation by a local, western-trained physician who practised classical homeopathy and Ayurvedic medicine. That physician is the healer responsible not only for getting me on the path to whole health but also for introducing me to Edward Bach and his thirty-eight powerful flower remedies. To put it mildly, my initiation into Edward Bach's world and his work was a major turning-point and one I didn't see coming.

After three years of study that included traditional graduate school and my recognition as a Registered Bach Flower Practitioner with the Dr Edward Bach Centre, I spent the next fifteen years in private practice, giving workshops in the US and the UK, as well as working as a US Retail Educator for Nelsons, the company responsible for distributing the remedies. During this time, however, I never lost my interest in the study of astrology, which went back to my late teenage years. In 2009, I added yet another layer to my education in this tradition; I entered an apprenticeship with Steven Forrest, one of the world's most respected Evolutionary Astrologers – a relationship which continues to this day along with my private practice, which is global.

In 2011, after establishing my practice in Evolutionary Astrology, I soon realized that in trying to maintain two such practices, plus travel for Nelsons and having a family life, something had to go. Although I turned my sole focus to Evolutionary Astrology, Dr Bach's work remains with me to this day, and that brings me to say a few words regarding his work.

It's been seventeen years since my first book, IGNITING SOUL FIRE: SPIRITUAL DIMENSIONS OF THE BACH FLOWER REMEDIES, was released, and yet very little has changed with regard to the application of Bach's wisdom and brilliance, explored in those pages. What wasn't explored at any length in IGNITING was Bach's interest in astrology. Even though very little is written about this, the subject has always intrigued me since I first started my journey with his work all those years ago. As a result, in the pages ahead you'll find an expansion of Bach's view on the astrological significance of our natal Moon and its karmic importance to our soul's discovery of purpose this lifetime.

As for his remedies in particular, if Bach were with us today, the global breadth his work has reached in the last ninety-plus years would astonish him, I think. Now, in this twenty-first century, there are several major flower-remedy repertoires around the globe. This doesn't count the thousands of people who prepare their own flower remedies from their gardens and the fields of nature, as Bach himself encouraged them to do. The fact that the discovery of flower-remedy therapy is universally acknowledged as exclusively his speaks for the brilliance of Bach's work. With such expansion have come many excellent resources to guide people throughout the world. They are examining his discoveries, studying his guidelines, and using the formulas and remedies in their daily lives. Several of these resources are listed in 'Further Reading'.

It's important to make clear that this book is not another manual to be placed alongside these resources. Readers already familiar with Bach's thirty-eight remedies will notice I've not included an examination of the Seven Helpers, nor have I included all the Final Nineteen remedies as application examples.

However, in the astrological chapters which discuss the lower expressions of the Moon by zodiacal sign and South Node (I'll explain that when we get there), you'll find clues to remedies in the descriptive text. And in the chapter discussing the South Node's emotional energy, I have included some remedies as 'suggestions.'

All in all, the pages ahead suggest ways for you to explore and discover the evolutionary path that's unique for you – with the help of Bach's philosophy behind his remedies, the self-knowledge held by your natal chart through the lens of Evolutionary Astrology, and the energy of your chakra centers.

On a final note, some relevant practical matters need explanation, regarding the visual style and some metaphorical images used within the text. As is the nature of books when they're taking shape, one of the challenges is the cover, the very first thing a reader sees and often a deciding factor of whether to pull it off the shelf. This book was no exception; it needed a cover that would convey the symbolic integration of Dr Bach's philosophy, the flowers, Evolutionary Astrology, and of course the energy of the chakras. Quite a tall order. As is the disposition with mind/body/

spirit projects, many things just present themselves, and so it was with this cover. The image of the zodiac, overlaid by expanding energy of a stylized flower and then the shafts of chakra energy reaching to the heavens, seems to say what needs to be conveyed. And then came the dragons. Again.

The little visual dragons, a creation of the artist, Morgan Hesmondhalgh, were a big part of the original IGNITING material, and with this new book they refused to be ignored. So what can one do? Using them as a symbolic metaphor for our difficult emotions throughout was here to stay, since Bach himself referred to the 'dragon of fear', a phrase I quote in the Afterword, which is a section written after the main text was finished. As a result, the editorial decision was made to keep the little imps from IGNITING as a primary visual imagery. As visuals, if nothing else, they are there to remind us of our necessary work as we travel on our evolutionary journey.

A few remarks on syntax and vocabulary used in the pages that follow are also necessary. In Bach's day, attention to being politically correct regarding gender specifics in writing and speaking simply did not happen. Today, of course, there is a great deal of attention paid to such details. In order to enhance the flow of thought, I've not attempted to insert notations such as 'he/she' in Bach's quotes or references to them. I felt this would be cumbersome and detract from the more important concepts. Thus, it should be understood by the reader that any reference to 'he' includes the feminine as well. This perspective also applies to the term, 'brotherhood'. Clearly, whether you subscribe to the camp that believes humanity is already a card-carrying member of the Aquarian Age or you're in the camp preparing for its arrival, more than ever this term includes the universality of all of us in human form, regardless of gender.

There is little doubt that Bach's gift as a healer and his

discovery of the remedies were divinely originated. Daily life on this planet has changed tremendously for most of us since Bach's death, especially during the writing of this book against the turbulent backdrop of the Covid-19 pandemic and political rhetoric.

Over the years, as noted, many have expanded his original thirty-eight remedies into larger systems with suggestions to the effect that Bach's work is out of date or out of touch with the times. This rationale would have us believe we live in a world climate far different from Edward Bach's and that, as a result, we have many more challenges emotionally. There are also the proposals that our energetic vibrations are shifting at a faster rate than Bach could have imagined. While I don't dispute that we are indeed living in very different times, we are still human, and the emotions of the human condition have not evolved into something new. Instead, we now find that difficult emotions occur with more frequency and at a higher level of intensity amid the landscape we have to navigate.

The circumstances creating such experiences are complex. We live in a world where our ecology, our security and, so recently, our health are all under constant threat. While many in the world are suffering from hunger, the rest of us who are well-fed are at risk nutritionally owing to the damaging ways our food supply is manipulated. In addition to the emotional stresses of our external environment, especially with the Covid-19 pandemic, many of us lack proper nutrition, which results in the body chemistry creating emotional roller-coaster rides. Despite passaging time, the range of our emotions is the same today as it was in Dr Bach's era: we are at times terrified; we become depressed or angry; we exhibit rage, and we experience detachment, joy, grief, and loneliness.

Bach was a healer who recognized that divinity or a Divine Spark exists in each of us. His intent was to make us aware of this divinity and to teach us further about the gentle divinity of nature and its ability to heal. His beliefs are steeped in simplicity, for in simplicity we find truth. Living in the age of speed and technology, we sometimes forget that we create a picture so complex that the simple solutions evade us.

Bach knew others would follow him in their attempts to 'improve' upon his work:

> *As soon as a teacher has given his work to the world, a contorted version of the same must arise.... [This version] must be raised for people to be able to choose between the gold and the dross.*

With the Age of Aquarius and its energy upon us, many of us find that we're compelled to explore our own spirituality and meaning for this lifetime. The questions before us are 'How can we heal our karmic mis-steps?' and 'How can we at the same time discover our own divinity in the quest for universal brotherhood/sisterhood?'.

This book delves deeply into Bach's own nature as a mystic and his gift as a healer, which was so much a part of him. The pages that follow are an exploration of the relationship between the deeper aspects of the remedies and their ability to help us find our high truth. In addition, if we embrace our astrological birth chart as our soul's blueprint for this lifetime with, as Bach proposed, its all-important Moon and the positive energy available in our chakras, we're primed to discover our soul's evolutionary purpose.

Bach was very clear and determined in following his own soul path, despite the difficulties it posed. I hope the pages before you will encourage you to open your heart to your own healing and, at the very least, kindle the flames of inspiration waiting to be discovered in your own soul. In this effort, I have endeavoured to show how deeply spiritual and introspective Bach's thoughts and writings were. It's important to remember that each moment of breath is an opportunity. What we choose in that moment is that which determines our next step.

TWO

—

Spiritual Law and Sacred Shopping

*We are a culture of spiritual seekers, closet mystics, and sacred
shoppers. But, you say, this culture has been around for eons. Well,
yes; but not like we see it today. The Age of Aquarius brings with it
energy that compels us to shift our personal energy to one that lives
the consciousness of universal brotherhood. Shift of consciousness is
the real news. This consciousness, for each of us, is a journey of our
emotions, of our Sacred Contract, forged between soul and spirit, for
the emotions are the gateway to the spiritual.*

I N ANCIENT astrology our spirit, the timeless Divine
Spark encased in the matter of the human body, was
symbolized as a dot within a circle, and this symbol is
still used by modern astrologers. Diversified esoteric teachings inform us that our spirit has engaged in a contract with
our soul and that a principle of this contract commands
we follow a path keenly orchestrated within a framework
of cosmic laws that can include *Rebirth, Karma, Opportunities,
Balance* and *Correspondence*. And it is on this journey that our
soul, our spiritual heart, holds continuous precise records
of our experiences and lessons; records available for us to
draw upon as a resource. If we use the laws of rebirth, karma, opportunities, balance and correspondence as our evolutionary resource, we have opportunities to develop depth
in our wisdom and can move forward in our growth. The
law of ***rebirth***, which is a core tenet of the evolutionary
astrological lens, determines that each of us remain in the

natural cycle of birth, death and earthly rebirth until that time when we attain a state of final transcendence beyond this cycle. This transcendence can only occur when we have completed our path of soul awareness and discovery of our personal High Truth and soul purpose.

So what is the catch? The catch is that it is through the body that we are compelled to learn our necessary soul lessons, for in order to discover our High Truth and soul purpose we must feel. In order to transcend and stop repeating the human life cycle, we need to be in the body so that we can experience all ranges of emotions and, thus, feel.

Spiritual teachings consider the soul to be the feminine aspect of the self. It is through this aspect that the Divine intends for us to connect with our emotional body. During each lifetime, the experience of our physicality brings us the extremes of joy and pain. It's through these emotional experiences that each one of us has the opportunity to access the feminine aspect we possess. Further, the range of emotions available to us brings value to our soul growth and self-empowerment.

Emotions are the key to developing our intuition, sometimes referred to as our 'sixth sense', which is a critical path of communication and understanding. If we step back and take a global view, it's easy to see that our attitudes of the past and the present not only affect our lives and the lives of others, but also that they have a direct correlation to the embryonic level of our awareness and sensitivity to this soul resource of intuition.

Within each lifetime, each one of us consciously and unconsciously experiences our emotional landscape, both externally and internally. These landscapes are in constant motion, are interactive, and profoundly affect how we function in the mundane world. More importantly, these emotional landscapes become a reflection of our relationship to Cosmic Law, challenging us to consider the consequences of not connecting to our emotional self.

The Law of **karma** purposely places us in circumstances and relationships within each incarnation whereby we sow and reap future consequences of emotional and physical interaction with others we've wronged or abused. Equally, we find that within each incarnation we again meet those whom we have loved or who have loved us. These are the encounters that bring us joy. More important for us, however, is to recognize that past wrongs can't be rectified, or joy in relationships appreciated, if we consciously cannot come to terms with our own emotions. Therefore, it's through these experiences and relationships that our soul propels us towards the awareness of what it means to feel.

Every situation or interaction with others requires a decision whether each of us will respond with malice or kindness, hate or love. Consciously or unconsciously, our emotional self drives these decisions. We can think of this particular law functioning like a set of karmic scales. How we respond to our internal and external environment through thought and action affects the balance of these scales and, thus, the direction of our future path.

In its divine wisdom, our soul provides circumstances for us in which we're presented not only with opportunities to pay off karmic debt but also to balance out this debt positively through love and kindness. This is the law of **opportunity**. Within the boundaries of this law, we're given freewill, but surprisingly, during our human experience, we take unexpected and unavoidable detours. The way we envisaged things would work out is not always the reality during this experience. We find that while we bask in the light of some achievements, more often than not the journey is fraught with disappointments and shattered dreams from unrealized expectations. The reason for this is that they aren't part of our soul's plan for us this lifetime. Two keys to our soul growth are found in both our reactions and actions to circumstances and life events. In other words, *our responses in thought and action influence the balance of our karmic scale.*

From a spiritual perspective, our soul is concerned with the concept of balance, and so it is that we're placed from lifetime to lifetime in environments that can vastly differ, swinging from one end of the spectrum to the other. For example, in one lifetime a person may find that life is easy and wealth accessible, and in the next they may be homeless. These lifetimes, however, composed of opposing elements, support us in the process of recognizing our emotional responses to life-events, in addition to the effect of our actions toward others. It's in this awareness as these lifetimes play out that we build up the resource of wisdom. This is the law of **balance**.

We now come to the fifth law, that of **correspondences**. This is the law which summarizes the basic principles of the other four. Healing is the balance of mind, body and spirit for others and for oneself through unconditional love. But working toward this state, even if we are aware of the goal, isn't easy. In its divine wisdom, our soul constantly sends us messages through these five cosmic laws within each lifetime. The problem is that when we don't get the message or see the opportunities, we can become fearful – frustrated and angry with what appears to be roadblocks surrounding us.

Driven to find answers amid our frustration, soul pressure, malcontent and other feelings, we become seekers, closet mystics, and sacred shoppers. We read, we practise postures, we meditate, and we pray. We study the stars and are inspired by psychics, rituals, and stones. We follow gurus and diets. We join circles and ashrams, never finding answers that seem to resonate with us; because in our frenetic search for the one thing that will point the way to our soul's intended purpose in this incarnation, our emotions become just as frenetic as our search. In our quest, we recall that some reference to exploring our emotional self has been made, but the idea of this excavation is put on the back burner. It seems too scary, or we may not like what we find. There are dragons down there. So in our anxiety we revert to where it's safe; the place where we believe we can maintain control of ourselves and everything around us: the mind.

In the past, when I lectured on Dr Bach and his work, I often used a metaphorical image of embarking on a spiritual journey, a pilgrimage of self-discovery. But this process often creates anxiety within us, and in this we're so afraid that we've missed out or taken a wrong turn, we never hear our soul whisper the key: *balance between our mind and emotions is the path to our high truth, our wisdom, and our soul purpose.* This is not an issue of heart versus mind. It's a matter of working in harmony, of learning to listen with the heart and then acting with the mind.

The divine universe works on a 'need to know' basis that's not in the business of giving us access to the complete picture. The lack of access to such trajectory vision is the divine plan for each of us, honed to perfection by a Divinity that never misses opportunities to humble us just when we think we know it all. In Native American mythology this cosmic posture is embodied in the coyote, otherwise identified as the 'trickster'. This rascal tricks us into believing we know the scheme and then playfully pulls the cosmic rug right out from under us. However, we do have an option, and it is this: we have to be willing to explore the emotions revealed to us – the unhealed conflicts within us – and be willing to participate in the transformation of our toxic patterns so that we can embrace our High Truth. This is what discovering our soul path is about. This is living on purpose. But living on purpose and the process of emotional discovery is a challenge in itself; and often we're not equipped to work alone. Being receptive to accepting help from those who can interpret, witness, and guide us is invaluable. Help of this sort worth considering may lie in various forms of therapy, including bodywork, art therapy, psychotherapy, or consulting a spiritual advisor.

In addition to these options, which are not exclusive ones, our resources should also include Dr Bach's Flower remedies. It is these 'God-sent Gift(s)' as Bach described them* that offer us a 'safety-net' as we explore our emotional self. Consideration of the remedies is important because once we have made this decision of self-examination, our journey can be a ride of emotional extremes. We find that our landscape varies between peacefulness and times of roaring through dark tunnels. In this darkness, we can't see; and it is in these moments that we want to abandon our intent, thinking we'll come back to 'it' another time. The difficulty is that once we have committed to this internal pilgrimage, our Contract ensures we must be present; we must take part in the process. There is no 'another time.' Our experiences, however, are only the wrapping paper enclosing the gift of the heart's wisdom. The Universe is clever, in that in order to access this wisdom held within the soul, our spiritual heart, we have to remove the outer wrappings. This process – and it is a process – is the alchemy of our journey.

Travelling along our path, our soul continues to whisper messages to us, but we find it difficult if not impossible to hear them, as we have a hard time surrendering our mental

*THE TWELVE HEALERS, p. 3

plan to our soul's plan. As we continue in our resistance, our external environment becomes difficult, forewarning us that we must shift our emotional perspective. Somehow, we don't get the message, and we ignore these warnings. Unheeded, these soul-messages begin to manifest in difficult life-events and/or relationships. Our emotions start to reel unpleasantly out of balance, and then it's only a matter of time before the body ceases to function in a balanced way.

The medical intuitive, Carolyn Myss, Ph.D., has a wonderful expression personifying this principle: 'your biography is your biology'. In other words, if we don't excavate our emotional distress and our karmic baggage, our body will reflect our resistance. For some of us, this means experiencing longer illnesses in order to learn necessary lessons for our soul growth. For others of us, the framework of these needed lessons may come in a combination of both external material and internal physical difficulties.

Another way of expressing this principle is to remember that whatever is happening to us internally will be mirrored in our external environment; the microcosm is a reflection of the macrocosm. *This is the Law of Correspondences.*

In those moments when we're brought to a state of crisis, whether it's emotional, physical, or both, they bring us to the edge of our personal abyss. THE TIBETAN BOOK OF LIVING AND DYING by Sogyal Rinpoche reminds us that to follow the path of our wisdom has never been more difficult; we do not live in a world that supports this. We live in a world that seems to be anchored in the mind, rather than the heart, and yet operating from the spiritual heart has never before been such an imperative.* The Aquarian energy we're coming into compels each of us to jump into our personal abyss, taking the leap of faith both as individuals and as the collec-

*THE TIBETAN BOOK OF LIVING AND DYING, p. 128

tive human race.

As we teeter on the edge of our abyss – not just once, but repeatedly – as we ignore our soul-messages, our fear and despair reflect the belief that we don't have operating instructions, maps or tools to manage the next right step. These beliefs, fuelled by the trickster, the crazymaker, create havoc anchored in our emotional body. In our fears and terrors, the ego tells us we're headed for disaster if we take the risk of embracing a leap of faith. The ego, fighting for control, doesn't recognize that we're in divine protective custody, and that in this custody, we have instructions, tools, and maps; we just have to learn how to recognize them where they rest in the wisdom of our spiritual heart.

Finally, the concept of chakras, established in the yogic tradition, is now widely accepted across most spiritual philosophies and by some practitioners of western medicine. For a diagram of them, see overleaf. These seven major centres of energy (and hundreds of minor ones) are mirrors of our emotional patterns reflected in a condition of expansion or contraction. Whether the emotional essence of a chakra is balanced (expanded) or unbalanced (contracted) has a direct effect on our physical state of wellness (or not). Dr Bach's remedies are powerful tools that can assist us in bringing to a place of balance in the chakras, and in doing so, they increase within us an awareness of soul messages through chakra patterns.

As we gain clarity in understanding the relationship between the emotional maps mirrored in our chakras and the balancing effect of the remedies, we can engage in bringing our body, mind, and spirit into harmony. The architecture of this process behind the discovery of our soul's intended path and high truth was *known* and well understood by Edward Bach, physician, healer … *mystic.*

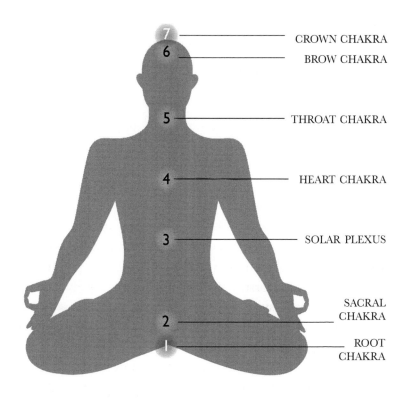

The Seven Major Chakras

THREE

—

Intuition is the Voice of the Soul

THERE'S A Buddhist expression ascribed to the fifth or sixth century teacher, Bodhidharma, that goes like this: 'All know the way, few actually walk it'. Listening to our intuition, our 'soul's voice', is part of walking the 'way'. Unfortunately, traditional society has only supported this concept by a weak acknowledgment that listening to our intuition (or gut, in some people's vocabulary) is a philosophy best left to the religious and business communities. At worst, traditionalists believe it's a malady of self-professed psychics and nutcases. For those of us who are not self-professed psychics and don't believe we are nutcases, learning to listen to our intuition is not only a tricky business; it can be a risky business. Each of us has a soul-job and none of us is here by accident, although sometimes we believe we are. Whatever the soul-agenda, it centres on transmuting karmic debt, taking it in, taking it on, inhaling it, and incorporating it into our soul growth. This takes us to a deeper, higher level of understanding, bringing us closer to home on our journey; recalling that we are spirit.

There are days when we can feel that the totality of our soul-mission is the job of self-healing, for the pain is so deep, there's no room or energy for anyone or anything else. Days like this are when we forget, if indeed we have ever learned, how to listen to our soul's voice, our intuition. This voice is there to guide us, particularly in times of extreme life challenges and lessons. It's also easy to assume that those who truly walk their intended soul path do so with some sort of special dispensation. This is simply not the case. We can look to Edward Bach as someone who not only knew the way, but who walked it despite disappointments, rejection, and obstacles.

Bach was one who clearly functioned within the framework of the five cosmic laws. Like the rest of us, he had no special dispensation. In fact, it was quite the opposite. He held the fierce belief that intuition is the voice of our soul. Not only did he know this philosophy, but he unquestionably lived it. A great deal of current research informs us that intent by the healer plays an important role in the therapy's effectiveness* and influence upon the intended individual. While we may feel bombarded with a plethora of choices in our sacred shopping, finding a truly gifted healer is difficult.

So what is a 'gifted healer?' Gifted healers use their intuition, natural skills, and knowledge with selfless intent and purpose to assist others in the discovery of their high truth through a balanced connection between their emotional mind and their intuitive heart. Certainly there's no doubt that Edward Bach was extraordinarily gifted, and someone who passionately believed that intuition and the voice of our soul are one and the same.†

Further, it's important for us to understand that Bach's spiritual beliefs and soul path are reflected in the discovery of the remedies. Keeping in mind that the mission of our evolution is to teach us how to feel, is it any wonder that the Bach Remedies are about this very thing; teaching us to

*Various forms of available therapies are outlined in MAKING COMPLEMENTARY THERAPIES WORK FOR YOU. Gaye Mack, 2007 (Polair Publishing, London)

†ORIGINAL WRITINGS, ed. Howard and Ramsell, p. 44

participate, reflect upon and embrace our emotions through opportunities that invite us to transform toxic patterns from our past? And in this process we just may discover our intended path for this life.

A great many books are available informing us about Bach's career as an orthodox physician and the course of events leading to his ground-breaking discovery of the Remedies between 1928 and 1935. Unfortunately, material is scant that extensively details his interest in matters of the esoteric or his explicit personal and spiritual connection to the plants and their resulting remedies. As the authority Julian Barnard points out, this lack of information may be due in part to the fact that Bach was most probably very private in such matters.* But, despite this deficiency, we can glean some insights about him. Though they lack specific details, Bach's two small books, HEAL THYSELF and THE TWELVE HEALERS (which relate exclusively to the remedies), express his spiritual philosophy within a broader framework.

The author Nora Weeks, who worked closely with Bach during the remedy years (1928–1935), wrote two books about him and his work. Although she clearly preserves an untarnished portrait of the man whom she so obviously respected professionally and personally, there is a lack of information over some personal details. For example, there's no mention of any personal relationships Bach had, other than professional ones. Although Weeks does tell us that Bach was a committed Freemason, believed in past lives, astrology, and other esoteric subjects, yet, unfortunately, more tellingy details simply are not forthcoming from her. In all fairness, however, we'd have even less knowledge about him if it were not for Nora Weeks. Following Bach's death in the autumn of 1936, along with the small group of supporters

*Barnard, 2002

who had assisted him during the remedy years, Weeks carried on the work at Mount Vernon (today known as the Dr Bach Centre) in accordance with Bach's request.

As a young radiographer, she left London with Bach in 1930 as his assistant when he abandoned orthodox medicine in pursuit of discovering a simple and pure system of healing. In her book, THE MEDICAL DISCOVERIES OF EDWARD BACH, PHYSICIAN, Weeks relates details of Bach's story as a physician and his discovery of the Remedies.

From the time of his youth, Bach *knew* that his destiny was that of a healer; it was just a question of whether he would seek his future through medicine or the church. Fortunately for us, he chose medicine, obtaining the combined diplomas of M.R.C.S. and L.R.C.P. in 1912, followed by the degrees of M.B., B.S. (1913) and D.P.H. (Cambridge, 1913). During his years in London as a medical man, his reputation grew so much that he was dividing his time between his consulting practice on Harley Street and his research laboratory at Park Crescent. By 1928, Edward Bach had come to a point in his professional career where he was recognized and honoured with distinction, both in the UK and abroad, for his work in bacteriology, immunology, pathology, and finally homeopathy.

However, there was another side to him, and it is here the story becomes intriguing. Even as a very young man, Bach was a keen observer of human nature, and he seemed to possess a highly developed intuitive sense about the suppressed emotional states of those around him. In his later years as a physician, this 'sense' extended to an awareness of obscured physical imbalances in others. Today, he surely would be regarded as a medical intuitive and empath. While his success as an orthodox physician and man of science grew in traditional circles, a major shift occurred in his experience with medicine in the later 1920s that had tremendous impact on the direction his life was to take.

Weeks relates that at this point he'd become increasingly dissatisfied with the methods used by those who practised traditional medicine. Privately, as a student of the esoteric, healing for him had become something other than a matter of treating the symptomology of illness or disease. For Bach, it was a matter of treating soul and spirit as well. In observing his patients, he recognized there was a definite connection between their emotional states and their chronic illnesses.

These observations led him to formulate his theory on the origins of illness and disease in the light of his belief that they resulted from a disharmony between the soul and the personality. Further, he was adamant that the method of regaining wellness came through harmonizing this disharmony. In fact, integrating the soul and the personality was the key to avoiding illness altogether. It also convinced him that nature held the keys to attaining this harmony. It was as if, in addition to what knowledge he had of the esoteric, he *intuitively knew* that the soul's message is to teach us how to feel. Through this process of both painful and joyful emotions, we develop our intuitive sixth sense, the voice of our soul. It would appear that this conscious awareness of the relationship between the soul and the personality was an indication of Bach's own expanding awareness and the soul path intended for him.

If we consider what we know of his personal history within the context of the Five Cosmic Laws, it's possible to get a glimpse of the path intended for him by his soul. This consideration is important. Bearing in mind that intention by a healer has a direct impact upon the healing process, consideration of Bach's intent and spiritual orientation is valuable in understanding the simple but profound healing potential provided by the remedies. Interestingly, just as it's useful for us to consider the framework of Bach and his work from a unique perspective, there is a core purpose to his remedies. They work to shift our emotional perception or framework so that we may realize our own path of purpose in this lifetime.

If we reflect on some of Bach's personality characteristics, we can additionally see how the laws of *rebirth, karma, opportunity, balances and correspondences* played out in his life. For example, as a young man, the city environment was very difficult for him. His state of health was always an issue, manifesting from minor to extreme life-threatening circumstances throughout his life until his death at the early age of fifty. Nora Weeks' accounts of Bach's personality relate his intense dislike of the city environment, and his constant struggle with a fragile central nervous system that was only soothed by the natural environment. Such nervous systems aren't unusual in those gifted with a heightened intuitive nature – such as psychics, including those with the gift of clairvoyance or ability to see images or visions.

We know from material available that he suffered chronic physical ailments in the early years of his medical career, and particularly during the years he worked exclusively with the remedies (1928–1935). Weeks reports him as saying to her, 'Are you ever unconscious of your body?' When she replied, 'Yes', he continued by saying, 'You do not know how fortunate you are. All my life my body has suffered in some way from pain and discomfort and distress.… I must know what pain is like and experience every kind to have a true understanding of what others suffer.'*

After the initial discovery of the first nineteen remedies in the repertoire, from 1928 to 1933, Bach went on to dis-

*ORIGINAL WRITINGS, ed. Howard and Ramsell, pp 180-1

cover the final nineteen in 1934 and 1935. This latter period was extremely difficult for him, both emotionally and physically. Prior to the discovery of a new remedy during this time, he would experience episodes that were debilitating physically and emotionally, according to Weeks:

> *For many days during the hottest period of the summer his body was completely covered by a virulent rash which burned and irritated incessantly; and for some weeks his legs were ulcerated, raw from knee to ankle; his hair came out and his sight almost failed. Before the finding of another remedy, his face was swollen and extremely painful. A severe haemorrhage exhausted him and the bleeding did not cease until the remedy for the mental state he was passing through was found.†*

Despite the precarious nature of his health, professionally and personally, Bach was a man whom we would describe today as a workaholic. This pattern was one that was not only evident during his years of medical study but stayed with him until he announced in 1935 that his work with the remedies was complete. While this behaviour of overwork severely taxed his health, this pattern and cost were most likely inevitable from an evolutionary perspective. Interestingly, but not surprisingly, we find similar patterns and constitutions in gifted healers within all cultures and traditions.

Bach, however, found relief for mind, body and soul in the countryside's freedom. To him, nature was Divine. He believed his highly developed intuitive sense in working with patients and the healing qualities and vibrations of the remedies were a divine gift of nature. His words reflect his humility, for he never referred to the remedies or their discovery as uniquely his. Rather, he viewed himself simply as a channel or conduit for:

*Weeks, MEDICAL DISCOVERIES, p. 116

Those Herbs of the field placed for Healing, by comforting, by soothing, by relieving our cares, our anxieties, [bringing] us nearer to the Divinity within. And it is that increase of the Divinity within which heals us ... thus we can truly say that certain Herbs have been placed for us by Divine Means, and the help which they give to us, not only heals our bodies, but brings into our lives, our characters, attributes of our Divinity. *

We can see the laws of rebirth and karma at work in Bach's recollection of past incarnations. In these recollections, he said he had always been a healer, although Nora Weeks notes these memories meant little to him. Seemingly, he was more concerned with the work he had come back to accomplish, knowing his work with the remedies could be passed onto others. However, his particular gifts of healing and 'sight', which he also acknowledged, were, as he put it, 'in higher hands' and could not be passed on to others.* Considering that he spent many past lives as a healer, we can surmise that his karmic mission in this life involved the task of providing all human beings with tools for their own self-healing. We know from esoteric writings that humanity through the ages has been given healing tools that far exceed our current knowledge and application. However, because of power struggles and abuse, they have 'gone underground' until such time as rediscovery has become possible and is used honourably.

Nora Weeks, in the passage mentioned earlier, briefly discusses Bach's esoteric interests and that he was a Freemason, but she doesn't detail much beyond this other than his affection for his Masonic brothers and his recollection of past lives as a healer. Julian Barnard however suggests that Bach's esoteric interests covered a far larger sphere, particu-

*Masonic Lecture, 1936, in Barnard, COLLECTED WRITINGS, p. 13

larly when it came to astrology. Apparently he originally felt that the distinctiveness of each of the Twelve Great Healers (the first twelve remedies) was unique because of the influence of the twelve signs of the zodiac.* In addition to his interest in astrology, it appears that he embraced the teachings of the Lord Buddha, Christ, and the Great Masters.†

Clearly, Bach worked and wrote within a metaphysical framework of his own determination. Further evidence of this is unmistakable in his reference to the collective of evolved souls known in metaphysical spirituality as the 'White Brotherhood'. In a letter written to a 'Brother' (presumably a fellow Mason) in 1934, Bach describes his anxiety for the future and that while lying 'near the tow-path at Marlow-on-Thames' a 'message came through'. He explains this message was not only for himself but also for all of those 'who are striving to help'. It is at this moment he comprehends the brilliance of a gorse bush within his sight. He adds to his comments that the Gorse remedy was the first of the Four Helpers. (Bach's Gorse remedy is recommended for hopelessness). Bach concludes his letter by stating that this experience would mean nothing to many people, but to him it showed how 'the White Brotherhood work, amongst us, not by miracles, not by apparitions, but by just leading us, if we are willing to be led, by every-day affairs'.§ While such metaphysical depths governed Bach's personal philosophy, Barnard accurately states that 'not everyone will continue with him on the journey'.¶ Nevertheless, his remedies are powerful regardless of one's personal philosophy.

Bach's break with orthodox medicine is not only evidence of his belief in the significance of listening to one's

*Barnard, COLLECTED WRITINGS, pp 77-8
†Barnard, 2002, p. 29   §ORIGINAL WRITINGS, p. 92
¶Barnard, 2002, p. 78

intuition; additionally, it was the very embodiment of the law of opportunity. With his interest in the wider scope of esoteric philosophy, there can be little doubt that Bach saw his departure from orthodox medicine as an opportunity to pay off old karmic debts. Further, of great importance, is that it gave him the opening to envision the larger picture of healing humanity through nature. He was aware as well this did not mean a 'free ride'. He viewed openings from the spiritual perspective, in that they often appear to us cloaked in difficulties and obstacles. Yet they are always for good reason:

> *Interferences occur in every life, they are part of the Divine Plan: they are necessary so that we can learn to stand up to them: in fact, we can look upon them as really useful opponents, merely there to help us gain in strength and realize our Divinity and our invincibility ... the more apparent difficulties in our path we may be certain that our mission is worthwhile.* *

Recalling that Bach based the keystone of his theory of illness and disease upon the concept of conflicts between the soul and personality (or mind), we can see that he virtually brings to our attention the essence of the law of balance in his remedies and likewise, the consequence of imbalance. His guide for healing was found in the balance of nature. In one account, Weeks refers to Bach being 'shown' the remedies. She cites that on one particular occasion, when he was in a mood that was withdrawn and aloof, he suddenly announced they needed to go in search of the flower to help this state. Upon finding 'water violet' Bach simply placed his hand over the flower and 'felt' what we might understand as a symbiotic resonance bringing him to 'a sense of peace, calmness, and humility.'*

*ORIGINAL WRITINGS, ed. Howard & Ramsell, p. 45: 'Free Thyself'

Barnard refers to these occasions as inner teachings, but regardless of the language, it's clear that Bach had a rapport with nature that was in concert with his soul.† He recognized that the life force of certain flowers had the ability to balance out specific distressful and toxic emotions, so that we may 'never know disease or illness'. If we step back a moment and consider Bach's intent through his work, we can see that he was a man who constantly sought a state of balance in all things and believed that the key to finding this was listening to our intuition.

Sadly, it seems, we find the law of correspondences mirrored in his lifelong struggle with his health. It's ironic that despite his genius and extraordinary gift as a healer, his own health was his nemesis. Bach's entire theory of illness and disease reflects this law; if we cannot reconcile internal toxic emotions, and repair the disconnection between mind and soul, the body will eventually break down. 'We each have a Divine mission in this world, and our souls use our minds and bodies as instruments to do this work, so that when all three are working in unison the result is perfect health and perfect happiness.'§

It's difficult to grasp why good health eluded him. It's harder still to believe that the causes of death listed on his death certificate were sarcoma (cancer) and cardiac arrest.¶ Louise Hay, in YOU CAN HEAL YOUR LIFE, ascribes cancer to deep unresolved pain and grief, carrying deep hurts. Carolyn Myss, in ANATOMY OF THE SPIRIT, cites numerous physical imbalances as they relate to the chakras and their emotional patterns. We can only surmise that in this lifetime Edward Bach was repaying enormous karmic debt on many levels. It's unfortunate that his profession, which at one time had

*Barnard, 2002, p. 36-7   †ibid., p. 36
§ORIGINAL WRITINGS, p. 41   ¶Barnard, 2002, p. 307

so honoured and respected him, abandoned him in the end when he began to speak his truth. Even more ironic is that if he practised today, he'd be respected as a brilliant mind/body physician in psychoneuroimmunology.

Bach was a man who didn't view life through a tunnel but envisioned the entire universe. Whatever he learned, it was never enough. He concluded in 1935 that for this lifetime his work was finished: with a knowing that his time in this incarnation was coming to a close in the fall of 1936. He wrote of this to a friend in that he was expecting 'a call to a work more congenial than of this very difficult world'.* His gift to us is this beautiful system of healing and the teachings that encourage us to listen to our soul through our intuition. In all of his humility, his burning desire was to leave all human beings with a way to heal themselves. It's doubtful he ever saw himself as the deep mystic he was. In the next chapter we take a look at the broad spectrum of what actually defines someone as a mystic in both the sacred and secular world and why we can identify Bach as one.

*ORIGINAL WRITINGS, ed. Howard and Ramsell, p.173. We shall return to this letter and its context in the Afterword to this book (see p. 209)

FOUR

From Medicine Man to Mystic

A S WE REVIEW our sacred shopping list of practices and philosophies that might reveal our soul's intention for us, we find a plethora of shamans, psychics, channels for sentient beings from the other side, clairvoyants, clairaudients, seers, and – yes – mystics. As I discussed in IGNITING SOUL FIRE, while some are sincere pilgrims, sadly, others are ill-advised charlatans. Thus, on our quest, discrimination is an important tool to have at hand, with the bottom line being, how do we know? *What qualifies one as a mystic?* How do we know Edward Bach was one? What exactly are the prerequisites for mystic status? Are only saints qualified for this lofty-sounding mantle, or is one a mystic first, then a saint? This question is relevant, because it gives us the opportunity to learn through Bach's personal history and his work with the remedies why he understood the relationship of suffering and solitude to spiritual growth and the soul's evolutionary purpose. While lots of suffering and solitude often shows up in discussions of mysticism, these are not always prerequisites. Portraying someone as a mystic (and in some cases, believing oneself a mystic) is all too familiar these days. Therefore, because of this rush to reverence, definition of mystical characteristics is significant in our understanding of why we can identify Bach as a mystic.

While over the years several authors have written about

the characteristics that identify a mystic, fortunately we have Wayne Teasdale's more or less contemporary account, THE MYSTIC HEART, published in 1999.* In his work, Teasdale addresses the subjects of mysticism, mystic characteristics, and the mystic path, which is particularly relevant to Bach.

According to Teasdale, the mystical pilgrim experiences distinctive states of consciousness and ways of being. And the path is one that is practical and actively experiential. The mystic takes part in their process in a way beneficial to their ongoing soul growth. This aspect can feel familiar to us when we work with Bach's remedies, as the remedies themselves gently prompt us to engage in participation and reflection that is governed by an intimate awareness of our own process.

For Teasdale, a mystic *lives* his–her path in contact with what is ultimately real; he or she doesn't just *talk about* it. This is another way of reiterating Bodhidharma's 'all know the way, few walk it' (see Chapter Three). However, like the singular mystical experience, there are moments of awareness that lack sufficient descriptive language, but are implicit through a different way of knowing. Furthermore, this 'knowing' that the mystic experiences is one that's noetic, giving one 'direct knowledge of the ultimate reality or the Divine ... a tasting knowledge of God'†

In this experience, there's an illumination of a universal connection between the temporal and cosmic world that doesn't require proof or explanation; it's integrative, absolute ... it simply is. Finally, Teasdale tells us that mystic

---

*In IGNITING SOUL FIRE: SPIRITUAL DIMENSIONS OF THE BACH FLOWER REMEDIES I include additional discussions on mystical characteristics according to author Evelyn Underhill, the American psychologist and philosopher William James and Barbara Dossey, R.N., Ph.D.

†Teasdale, p. 23

spirituality is a practical, spiritual wisdom. Within this wisdom there's a particular knowledge of cosmic law and its process. The intuitive knowledge of this wisdom connects to the Divine at deep levels, and for some there is the added gift of sensing the emotions and motives of others on their own journey.

The path that the mystic treads manifests in many forms, expressions and traditions. By referring to these characteristics as touchstones, we have the opportunity to weed out any charlatans lurking in our own particular bushes. At the same time, we can come to understand why Bach is rightly called a mystic.

Spiritual teachings, teachers, and scholars identify characteristics that are broadly applied across many traditions and philosophies. However, because there are countless portrayals of mystics through the ages, we find there's a collage that cuts across boundaries both sacred and secular alike. Mystical characteristics are to some extent subjective. Therefore, not all 'mystics' will adhere to a precise list of identifiers, nor do all mystics exhibit mystical characteristics in the same fashion.

Many people believe they have had at least one mystical experience in their lives. Mystical profiles from the past provide us with an interesting mixture of characteristics described by Teasdale and others. The mix includes both balanced and unbalanced aspects of a life that brought them face to face with difficult relationships. Many had a skewed sense of self and doubted their abilities. While these struggles were part of their fabric, in mystics there seems to be an overriding motivation that is or was a burning desire to achieve direct knowledge of the Divine, both internally and externally. It's a combination of such characteristics that propelled them onto their mystic path.

Just as the mystical path can manifest through various behaviours, the initial mystical awakening can occur in a variety of ways. It can happen through a singular event, or it may unfold through a process culminating in an eventual awareness of internal conflict with the external environment.

Teasdale states that 'each of us is called to be a mystic'.* This is most definitely a surprise. It's a surprise in that each of us has such potential. It affords us, as well, the opportunity to perceive Bach in an entirely different light. In this, we have yet another surprise. This new perspective becomes important to our ability to embrace the core messages his flower remedies hold for our souls and the roles they play in helping us manifest our highest purpose in this incarnation. As seekers, we are in a process of initiation that requires we travel down into the inner self. This is not an exercise of the head and mind that gravitates toward rationalization.

For this reason, the journey is not an easy one. Being called to the mystic path, our soul path becomes one of a series of initiations. Initiations are:

> *An expansion of consciousness to a realization of the all-ness and completeness and universality of God's love. That expansion of consciousness or initiation comes when you can ... hold fast to faith – even if it seems that all you have worked and stood for, all you believe in and hope for, crashes and crumbles about you. Now is the very limit of your test, and your initiation is at hand.... When you are pushed to the very last degree of endurance, the light breaks for you and you know that all you have stood for and held to is eternal truth.†*

In other words, initiations are not meant to be easy.

In exploring Bach from this perspective, we can discover

*Teasdale, p. 119
†White Eagle, in *Stella Polaris*, 1952-3, p. 184

the essence of this man beyond his gifts as a brilliant physician. Leaping into the fresh territory, we have the opportunity to witness an expression of absolute and contemporary mysticism and in the process perhaps discover mystical characteristics within ourselves.

A pattern that seems to appear with most mystics is that they disconnect, in a sense, from a life that has been familiar. How and when this disconnection takes place varies individually. For many, the driving force is an inner struggle between the incessant chatter of the rational mind and listening to the voice of the soul. As Bach began his work with the remedies, he identified this conflict as the cause of illness and disease.

Bach's obsession with work, not unlike the behavioural patterns of other mystics, clearly intensified the chronic fragility of his health. He added further demands upon himself when he chose to live a simple life after he left London. At first glance, the decision would seem to have been a supportive one in view of his other behaviours. However, this was not the case. His choice led to very difficult circumstances, far different from the financial freedom he'd enjoyed through his consulting practice in London. When he and Nora Weeks left London to continue and expand the work with the remedies, Bach refused to charge patients for his services. As a result, his resources were chronically scarce: so much so that when they settled at Mount Vernon (the Bach Centre today), Bach had to make most of the furniture for his consulting rooms himself.*

Solitude is an environment most mystics crave, and in this Bach was no exception. His relationships (both personal and professional) seemed to fluctuate. While Nora Weeks reports he liked to go to the pub for a singsong and a few

*Weeks, DISCOVERIES, p. 111

pints with the lads, information regarding close friends away from his work is not available from her writing. During his marriage to his first wife, Bach fathered a child by another woman, whom he later married after his first wife died of diphtheria. He separated from his second wife in 1922.*

Clearly, Bach was an enigma. Both Weeks and others describe him as a man who could be blunt, impatient, and yet unendingly compassionate. Weeks comments that while he had a keen interest in village affairs, he needed unending time to be alone and to walk the countryside. Progressively abandoned by the profession that had just a few years previously held him in the highest esteem, it seems the company he most preferred was that of his Masonic brothers and his few companions working with him in the remedy research.

The need for solitude among those on the mystic path, such as Bach, is a double-edged sword. Solitude can evolve into intense loneliness and crisis of spirit as the person becomes faced with his or her own dragons, and the abyss. Aside from grappling with the mystic's emblematic characteristics of chronic health problems, difficult relationships, the desire for simplicity of life, and the experience of intense loneliness, it is Bach's unique rapport with nature that underscores the fact of his walking the path of a natural or nature mystic.

The Divine has produced many natural or 'nature mystics', according to Teasdale – who has quite a lot to say about their characteristics. As a group, nature mystics have an intrinsic connection to all of life through the natural world. For them there's an innate understanding of the symbology and messages nature freely offers to humankind. For the nature mystic this connection to the natural world is a 'reality [that] is revelational ... that trigger[s] higher states of awareness.'*

*Barnard, p. 305

There's an intimate relationship and, most importantly, a level of consciousness with the Divine through the natural world that simply does not resonate to such depths with others. Nature mystics express these dynamics through mediums such as the arts, ritual, writing, and the arts of medicine and healing. Edward Bach expressed his symbiotic relationship with nature and his service to humanity through the discovery of the remedies and his passionate desire that others freely learn how to use them for their wellbeing and discovery of soul purpose.

On the mystic path, there is no room for greed, arrogance, or over-concern with accruing substantial possessions as a means of identity or power. If these emotions become driving forces, the conscious awareness of and the connection to all life, along with the ability to feel the struggle and pain of others, is unattainable. Some pilgrims also possess the extraordinary gift of high sensitivity to the motives and emotional depths of others. Edward Bach is included in this group. Further on in the astrological discussion regarding his natal chart, we'll see that this identification isn't a coincidence. As his intuitive abilities became increasingly stronger, he had the ability to heal by touch and, occasionally, could foretell events. Weeks notes:

> *Through his finely developed sense of touch he was able to feel the vibrations and power emitted by any plant he wished to test; and so greatly was his body receptive to these vibrations that it reacted instantaneously. If he held the petal or bloom of some plant in the palm of his hand or placed it on his tongue, he would feel in his body the effects of the properties within that flower....†*

> *Bach's great compassion and links with all things and people formed a link between them and him, and by reason of this sympathy, he*

*Teasdale, p. 192   †Weeks, DISCOVERIES, p. 50

would hear the call for help from any in distress. *

This awareness is essential for aspiring mystics and for those of us attempting to discover our soul purpose. However, this doesn't mean there are not struggles, obstacles, and disillusionment along the way. According to Bach's friend and colleague, Dr F. J. Wheeler, 'the last seven years of his [Bach's] life were lonely ones for him; his work during that period was based entirely on the knowledge that he gained intuitively and for such, the world has little understanding or encouragement, needing causes, scientific provings, before it is ready to believe.'† From statements made in one of his last public appearances before his death, it's clear that Bach had found solace in and connection to the Divine through his work with the remedies. He said:

> *We carry a Spark of the Divine that within us resides a Vital and Immortal Principle. And the more that Spark of Divinity shines within us, the more our lives radiate its sympathy, its compassion and its love, the more we are beloved by our fellow-men.... From time immemorial, man has looked at two great sources for Healing. To his Maker, and to the Herbs of the field which his Maker has placed for the relief of those who suffer. Yet one Truth has mostly been forgotten. That those Herbs of the field placed for Healing, by comforting, by soothing, by relieving our cares, our anxieties, bring us nearer to the Divinity within. And it is that increase of the Divinity within which heals us.§*

Spiritual teachings stress, 'Humanity is one vast brotherhood of life ... all nature is part of you – you are part of nature'.¶ The portrait of Edward Bach as a mystic is one

---

*Weeks, DISCOVERIES, pp 106-7   †ibid., p. 139
§Masonic Lecture, 1936, in Barnard, COLLECTED WRITINGS
¶White Eagle, ON THE GREAT SPIRIT, p. 75

that brings into focus some compelling realities about the man. In our contemplation, we come to realize that were he alive today, his compassion would undeniably reach out to us. Whether physician or friend, acquaintance or not, he would sit beside us, hold our hand and encourage us through our distress. He would stand at our back as we face hard challenges and he would heal us with his insights, energy, and his remedies.

While Dr Bach is no longer with us, his messages are. Exploration of our emotions is a necessity for discovery of our soul's intended purpose for us if we're serious about travelling the mystical path. As was acknowledged back in Chapter Two, this exploration is a formidable challenge. Most of us will attempt to negotiate our way around what is actually a prerequisite for our work, convincing ourselves that confronting the dragons of our emotions is not only unnecessary, it promises very unpleasant experiences.

Nevertheless, this confrontation is essential. In the chapters that follow, we take a closer look at the ways in which our personal dragons manifest and how we can recognize and transform them from adversaries into elements of empowerment.

FIVE

—

Here be Dragons

MEDIEVAL cartographers had a common practice when mapping the world as they knew it. When the mapmaker had ascertained all he could from his storehouse of knowledge of geography, he would letter the phrase, 'Here be Dragons', across the void, thus creating a boundary between the safety of known territory, and the ominous abyss of the unknown beyond. Throughout our lifetime, the Divine pushes us through dark tunnels – and just when we think we may be seeing the light at the end, we emerge, only to find that we are looking into the abyss … where the dragons lurk. And yet, it's this confrontation of sorts that signals our initiation onto the mystic path in our quest to discover our evolutionary purpose.

The image of the dragon was a familiar one to the ancients, and in the present, it still is. The national symbol of Wales is the icon of a Red Dragon, while a moment's thought of the dragon also conjures up Scotland's eternally famous water dragon, 'Nessie'. Some sources of Welsh mythology connect dragons to the four elements of fire, earth, air, and water and for us as we travel on our journey, it's these elemental dragons of emotion that hold keys to our own unexplored territory, and in what follows I have given the dragons their Celtic names. In such lore, these dragons – Draig-Teine, Draig-Talamh, Draig-Athar and Draig-Uisge, are sometimes represented as the dragons of fire, earth, air and water respectively. This is the very territory we need to explore – the emotions of our primeval great deep. And, it's this excavation that will assist us in moving through the baptism of fire, earth, air, and water that moves us forward upon our soul path.

Draig-Teine*
I Am on Fire with Passion, Obsession and Pain

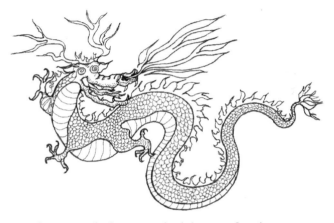

In astrology, mythology, and alchemy, fire is synonymous with energy, mastery and, most importantly, transmutation. The emotions of passion, obsession and pain in one way or another are emotions heralding our initiation through the element of fire. The Universe and everything within it works within a framework of polarities, including the realms of science and spirit. As both scientist and mystic, Edward Bach recognized the polarities of emotion in his patients and particularly within himself. The foundation of his work with the Remedies is built upon the realization that the negative state of our emotions fuels illness and disease, and that trading contraction for expansion is the only way to wholeness and growth. But, in order to shift our relationships with toxic emotions, which he knew only too well from his own life, we must be willing and have the courage to confront our emotional dragons head on.

For most of us, the emotion of passion conjures up positive images such as the pleasant feelings one experiences in the ardour of love or in enthusiasm for art or music. Years ago, when I was an undergraduate, a professor of mine in comparative religions made the statement, 'whatever your passion is, that which means the most to you, this is your religion'. For some time I never could understand his thought-process fully until I realized he was talking about emotion.

The emotion of passion in the positive sense is exciting and can take your breath away. The work toward a universal ideal often gives birth to passion because of the felt enthusiasm for the cause which, when balanced, creates leaders and teachers for the good of humanity. However, when the fire of such passion converts into the contracted negative state, it becomes so intense that the qualities of leadership and wisdom become zealous, willful, and inflexible, burning out the individual and those around them. Sadly, we see such passion all too vividly in the world today, passion in which the original spirit has become intangible and lost.

In our passion, anxiety appears. It can ratchet up to a state of obsession – which can make us believe we will never have enough, do enough, or be enough. In our perception that there will never be enough, we want and grasp for more. It is the need to feed the chronic wanting that drives this grasping within us, Buddhist psychologist Jack Kornfield comments – identifying it as our 'hungry ghost'.* If only we had more, could do more, we would *be* more. It's ironical that in our frenzied obsession to feed our ghost, we come to believe that the fire of our intensity will correspond to progress on our soul path. What we don't comprehend is that the fire of such emotional obsession burns so hot that it forestalls any movement forward on our path. This is

*Kornfield, A PATH WITH HEART, 1993

not the fire of positive emotions fuelling our soul purpose. Instead, the smoke from our obsessive fire dragon billows around us, preventing our ability to see the way forward. Unable to see or recognize that we shall never be able to fill our 'hungry ghost', our wanting continues out of control, whispering to us that we will never be satisfied. We never will have enough ... unless we can shift our perspective.

When we put our hands too close to the fire, we feel pain. A woman in labour, about to give birth, feels pain with the growing intensity of each contraction. Contraction brings pain, whether it's physical or emotional. From an emotional perspective, it can be some time before we experience the painful outcome of this fire; but when we do, it always comes with the strings of karmic law and the law of correspondences attached. The good news is that in the excavation of our emotional 'dig' we have the opportunity to engage the positive nature of the fire dragon, which can manifest as constructive energy and mastery. Above all, fire transmutes, purifies, and transforms ... and in spiritual law, **Love** is the elemental lesson of Fire.*

Draig-Talamh
I am bound to the Earth by Resistance, Indecision and Worldly Fears

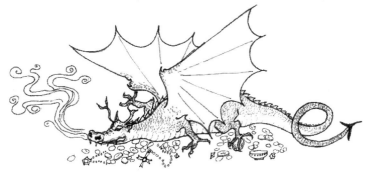

*White Eagle, THE PATH OF THE SOUL, pp 73-4

In spiritual teachings, esoteric writings and psychology, the reference to 'being grounded' (or ungrounded) often appears. Being 'grounded' or 'ungrounded', in these contexts, is a description of one's energetic or emotional state. Often it refers to both simultaneously. The inference here is that the grounded person is well-balanced emotionally and energetically, able to perceive his or her surrounding environment with clear perception. But as with all things, there can be too much of a good thing – and the element earth is no exception; we can be far too entrenched in it. The expression, 'earthbound' is not one that refers to a positive state of affairs. When seen in older writings, it refers to the soul or spirit of a dear, but expired, Aunt Petunia or Uncle Herald unable to ascend into the glory of the ethers.

As we proceed along our journey, our environment constantly changes, and there are times when we become excessively grounded in the element earth. Whether we're aware of it (and often we are just simply oblivious), we find ourselves at an impasse. Here the dragon of earth has captured us, manifesting as excessive resistance, indecision and/or fear.

If we reflect thoughtfully on the emotion of fear, it's easy to see that as a basic emotion it pushes the 'buttons' that ignite many secondary, contracted emotions that are part of the human condition. Recalling this emotional state of the fire dragon, we can easily see that fear is a primary emotion. The contracted experience of the element earth is no exception, although it appears through different expressions.

Emotional resistance is powerful and refers to a state of contraction that prevents us from 'hearing' valuable advice and urgings from those around us. But, far more important to our spiritual journey, resistance inhibits us from hearing critical messages from our soul. An axiom of spiritual law dictates that the more we resist, the harder the lesson. Furthermore, that which we resist the most is actually the thing we need to embrace. But do we listen? Of course not.

Evolutionary astrologers often look at the influence of such resistance through the placement of and aspects to the planets Saturn and Pluto in a chart. This can be quite significant in order to determine those areas of a person's life or behaviour that might prove disruptive to their soul growth. For the purposes of this discussion, our focus will be on Pluto. Astrologically, this planet is often referred to as 'the Transformer', or the 'Cosmic Two-by-four', in the sense of a heavy wooden joist. As we move along in our evolutionary journey, the Universe gives us many clues and opportunities to make both emotional and physical changes necessary in support of our progress. Unfortunately, we often continue on, believing we know better than anyone or anything how we should do this journey of ours, ignoring the messages. In a word, we 'resist'. When this happens,, there are almost always consequences in some manner.

In mythology, Pluto is the lord of the underworld, but astrologically, the planet's energy is psychological. Along with Pluto's placement in our birth chart, when transitting Pluto triggers a particular sensitivity in our chart, it's not unusual for us to feel deep emotional turmoil during the transit. The evolutionary intent here is about bringing whatever needs to be looked at up from the depths and into the light, so that we may move forward. A well-known quote from the psychologist Carl Jung on this process reads, 'One does not become enlightened by imagining figures of light, but by making the darkness conscious.'*

During a Pluto transit, in addition to emotional distress, the transit can manifest in the guise of external events that force us to make changes we previously ignored. Strange

*https://www.quotes.net/quote/43234

as it may seem, there appears to be a direct correlation between the extent of our resistance and the intensity of our particular experience. Sometimes we just do not get it until we're hit over the head and brought to our knees.

Indecision is a bedfellow of resistance. In our resistance, life doesn't fall into place as we think it should (because, remember, we aren't listening or paying attention), so we become full of self-doubt and eventually may move into a chronic state of indecisiveness. There's not one decision we can make with a steadfast mind and, as a result, we forever question ourselves, coming to a point wherein no decision is the decision.

Unlike some of our other emotions which possess positive attributes that balance their negative states, neither resistance nor indecisiveness have any positive value. Stuck in a place that has us trapped by them, there's no way we can move forward on our evolutionary path. As if resistance and indecision were not enough, the culprit often lurking behind these two states of being is fear of worldly things. These are the things Edward Bach described as the fears of everyday life.* If we're afraid of the dark, of illness, pain, being with others ... the world in general, is it any wonder that trapped in the clutches of the earth-dragon of worldly fears we become resistant and indecisive? Sadly, being irrationally afraid of the surrounding environment, and being resistant and indecisive, prevents us from being in the world. In this state it's difficult to reach out, to engage with others, or to connect with our soul purpose. In a phrase, we can't be of service, and the paradox in this is that the elemental lesson of earth is **Service**.

*Barnard, COLLECTED WRITINGS, p. 37

Draig-Athar

*I am suspended in Air from Restlessness,
Confusion and with Detachment*

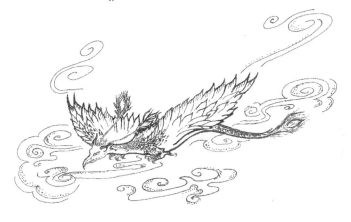

The element air is a metaphysical symbol for inspiration, insight and, in its highest expression, illumination. These are all characteristics of the mystic path, but for some of us, the fullest and most balanced expression of these markers is out of reach when we become mired in detachment, confusion and restlessness. It is in these states of non-awareness that we circumvent our soul's agenda for our journey.

We may recall that spiritual initiations are not meant to be easy, and cosmic law challenges us by propelling us out of our comfort zones. These 'opportunities' show up not once but frequently, pushing us into an uncharted space that shows up through a variety of manifestations. In these moments, when anxiety sets in and we lose our footing, the dragon of air takes up residence in the seat of our emotional self and life can become scary. The experience makes us feel as if we are flying at high altitudes, deprived of the oxygen to maintain our focus. In this space we panic, certain we're losing our way on the journey. Reactively, we grasp for safety in the mind, and in our anxiety and restlessness, we count on the rational brain taking over and getting things under control. This is an illusion.

The reality is that if we could acknowledge our denial concerning the true state of our emotions, we'd be able to admit that in fact we don't know who we are or where we really are going. However, since we cannot do this when we're in the clutches of the Air Dragon, we mask our disorientation by appearing indifferent and detached to the rest of the world. The difficulty is that we can't hold this space indefinitely because eventually our soul will shatter this illusion through chaos in one form or another.

Emotional betrayals leading to loss of faith within ourselves and with others are often the driving force behind personal chaos. The irony is that from the spiritual level, those who feel they've been betrayed and then lose faith are often the people who possess deep wisdom garnered from many lifetimes of experience and learning. And while they may sense something urging them to speak from deep within, there can be a vague sense of some unidentified trauma that keeps them from pursuing, much less expressing, this intuitive sense or soul-voice.

Since they can't specifically identify this vague sensation, they dismiss it and the struggle continues. The rational mind becomes insistent that they 'keep a lid on it', deferring any notions of intuition for the mind to sort out. For those caught up in this impasse, unable to trust, much less speak, their intuitive voice with confidence, the internal struggle intensifies and the wisdom held within the soul remains obscured. On the brink of emotional chaos, they seek refuge by detaching from the external environment and thus escape upwards into the ethers of the mind. From this space, there are essentially two ways of being. If the individual goes one way, he or she rationalizes everything, including his or her emotions, speaking of them as if they were being viewed under a microscope held at arms' length. In going the other way, he or she takes on the 'air' of being 'in the world, but not of it', in the negative sense.

From an energetic perspective, the inherent danger is that in either scenario, these individuals have become ungrounded. In this state, a door opens which invites an entirely alternative way of being in the world that isn't on the soul's agenda. Either they completely retreat into the perceived safety of introversion, or they develop a skewed sense of grandiose importance.

For those with illusions of grandeur, fantasies of extraordinary 'spiritual gifts' place them in an imagined position of power over those 'less-evolved'. The journey of the path, as the Buddhists say, is simple; 'chop wood, carry water'. But those who live in the realm of fantasy about themselves and their 'gifts' simply do not plug into the reality of the journey. Conversely, for those truly on a mystic path, like Edward Bach, the spiritual agenda really *is* to 'chop wood, carry water.' Sadly, in the Aquarian Age, we're so inundated with self-professed gurus, psychics, clairvoyants, shamans and mystics, that it's difficult to discern the wheat from the chaff. However, spiritual teachings tell us 'most major work is done quietly'.

Bach knew this as well. He pursued his work with the remedies without pretence and in a steadfast manner that did not engage fanfare or notoriety. His was a system of healing that he identified as 'simple and pure'.* So in our effort to travel our intended soul path, our progress becomes measured by our level of self-awareness and the ability to tap into and trust the innate wisdom of our soul-voice. When this happens, it brings with it moments of grounded

*ORIGINAL WRITINGS, ed. Howard and Ramsell, p.176

insight, inspiration and, ultimately, wise illumination that we're meant to share selflessly with others along the way. This is the soul's intent for each of us, for the lesson of the element Air is **Brotherhood**.

Draig-Uisge
I am drowning in the Waters of Fear, Anger and Grief

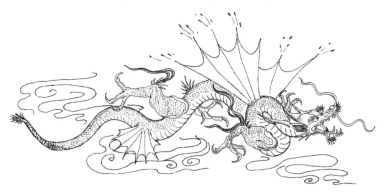

The element water, essential for all forms of life, 'creates, nourishes and destroys physical form … [it] is concerned with the soul of things – with the psychic aspect of our being, that part of us which senses, reflects, and absorbs the impressions of the world around us'.*

Classically, the element of water symbolizes emotions dwelling in the very root of our being. And, like a body of water, these emotions can be calm. Conversely, the water dragon of our emotions can spring up from the depths of our being, manifesting in emotions that churn, sending us out of control.

As a mystic who possessed the gift of being able to sense unspoken emotional states in others, Edward Bach himself felt the emotional dragons of fear, anger, and grief from those around him. In view of this, it's no coincidence that

*Joan Hodgson, ASTROLOGY, THE SACRED SCIENCE, p. 62

his earliest flower remedies were ones that address these particular negative emotional states.

When we experience our old nemesis, fear, in its positive manifestation, it functions as a necessary safety net: warning us of danger, cautioning us to stop so that we may reassess our situation, behaviour, or plan of action. However, irrational and unrestrained fear catapults us out of emotional balance, driving us into watery depths that can cause destructive behaviour and unwise choices. Fear of loss, the emotion that is one of our most intrinsic, can drive us into depression, non-action and disempowerment.

Unfortunately, there's no authentic spiritual philosophy that promises the journey of discovery to our soul's purpose will be easy. In fact, quite the opposite is true: facing our fears can be guaranteed to be a prerequisite for forward progress. Simply, there's no way around this one; either you face your fear or you don't. Spiritual teachings also tell us that if we dwell on those things we are most afraid of rather than face them, we'll draw them to ourselves in some form. In this, the soul's purpose is to give us the opportunity to transcend and transmute those fears. The only way to get to the other side of fear is to go through it. If we find that we're simply unable to master such opportunities in this lifetime, not to worry; the Universe can supply endless future occasions, for lifetimes to come. Such is the way of the laws of karma and rebirth.

Difficult as it is, the emotion holding the greatest power over us is psychological fear. While the path of the mystic includes service with each of us possessing this potential, fear is the one emotion that can abort our fulfilment of this destiny.

A familiar bedfellow of fear is the dragon of anger, for usually it's fear that fuels anger. Anger can bear many facets, including rage. While the experience of fear can have a beneficial effect, as in warning us of danger, there is no benefit to rageful or revengeful anger or the behaviour that it drives. 'In-your-face rage' is an all-too-common way of being these days, and one that has gone from a microcosmic framework into a macrocosmic explosion with terrifying global repercussions.

But anger is not always 'in-your-face rage'. The smouldering emotion of repressed anger is just as destructive. This emotional state can remain banked like the coals of a fire for years, ready to reignite at any given moment. Bach identified this type of anger as one that leads to resentment, self-pity and bitterness. As secondary emotions, they set the stage for the eternal victim who in his–her unrealized state of entitlement is merely another aborted mystic.

The emotional dragon of anger, whether rageful or repressed, harms others physically and psychologically. Eventually unresolved anger turns in on the self, destroying the cellular structure. The body can't tolerate this kind of pressure indefinitely. If these dragons aren't quelled through resolution and balance, the body will break down, bringing us to our knees in a heartbeat through illness or acute mental stress or distress. At this point we have the opportunity to find resolution and rebuild our health, or not. If not, the universe will give us more opportunities in the next incarnation. The choice is ours.

There is yet another water dragon that can drown us, and this is the dragon of grief. Grief involves the loss of anything dear to us, has provided safety to us, or has been a part of us. While it's a natural part of life, grief isn't an emotion our soul means us to experience perpetually on our path. The experience is meant to teach us the process of honouring and then letting go. This is part of our evolutionary growth. If we honour this progression by moving through it, we create space for the energy of new experiences and opportunities to present themselves. And it is in this constant movement that we experience exactly what our soul intends for us.

In her many writings and workshops, Caroline Myss often refers to those who become married to their grief as 'staying in their woundology'. When referring to former clients, I've heard her comment that they could stay in their woundology as long as they wished; she simply was not staying there with them. Myss' point here is that staying stuck in our grief is a guaranteed way to stay stuck in life and, therefore, stuck on our mystic path. This doesn't mean that we should not honour our grief as a necessary process of the human experience, but in order to make progress in discovering our soul purpose, we have to be willing to let go of it and move on. Nothing is indefinite in the human experience, and grief shouldn't be either. Grief is the messenger of change, and with change, there's opportunity. The issue is, how will we respond to our opportunities?

If we stay stuck in our fear, our anger, our rage or our grief, we have no chance of learning the elemental lesson of Water, which is **Peace**.

*

As we journey along our evolutionary path in search of our soul's intended purpose, it's a given that we will encounter the emotional dragons connected to fire, earth, air and water. But what we need to remember is that on our pilgrimage, our soul is whispering to us, cautioning us to pay attention, to be aware, to reflect and to participate in slaying our dragons. It's no coincidence that we'll meet these dragons again, but through the evolutionary astrological lens as we explore the importance of the Moon in our natal chart, which Edward Bach believed was so significant. First, however, we need to take a look the concept of his soul types/ personalities and their lessons.

SIX

—

Soul Type, Service and our Universal Connection

A S WE HAVE seen, Bach, as a mystic and student of the esoteric, strongly believed every one of us is Divine. And in our Divinity, each of us has a job to do in this lifetime in the name of service and brotherhood. Whether we achieve our goal in this lifetime is uncertain. What is certain is that according to cosmic law we're given plenty of opportunity for discovering our soul purpose, either in this incarnation or in future ones.

In earlier chapters, there was discussion regarding the mis-steps some people make in their desire to be spiritual. Ignoring the emotional excavations that must be a part of our evolution, some of us choose to focus upon our sacred shopping, anxiously obsessed that we will miss the mark. In making misguided choices through our obsessions and anxieties, we can become intransigent and dogmatic in our chosen beliefs and rituals in the name of spirituality. Unfortunately, in this mindset we may also take on the undesirable mantle of pious self-righteousness. The danger here is that this attitude can lead to unwarranted cruelty, judgment, or anger towards others who are far from deserving of the repercussions of such misguided emotions.

Spirituality is definitely not about piety or self-righteousness; it's about *service* and *universal connection*. By working the patterns of our own feelings and shifting those that are contracted into an expansive state, we can make the discovery within ourselves of our evolutionary purpose. This often manifests in the simplicity of desire to serve without expectation and in the understanding of what brotherhood truly means. In our contemporary world, the concept of brotherhood has taken on a more expansive meaning from Bach's time. While astrologers and astronomers differ as to whether or not we've technically entered the Aquarian age, there's no denying technology has shifted our planet into a global community of universal connections. With this comes the meaning of brotherhood from Bach's time as well as service, both of which are a characteristic of Aquarian energy.

In this understanding, Edward Bach was crystal-clear in his writings:

> *Impersonal service done, not even for spiritual promotion, but just for the desire to serve. This is the keynote of the hindrances you are now to investigate.* *

Patterns of numbers intrigued Bach, which isn't surprising as Freemasonry and astrology are rooted in mathematics. He maintained that the keys to transforming our 'emotional hindrances', so that we may access our spiritual self, rests in the spiritual heart of twelve distinct soul types or soul personalities. Alongside these soul types, he placed the first twelve of his remedies, those he identified as the Twelve Great Remedies', later calling them 'the Twelve Healers'.†

Clearly, while the universe may hold an infinite number of soul types, Bach chose not to tackle the prospect of such a massive field and instead opted to keep his work simple within the twelve. He also maintained that these twelve

---

*Barnard, COLLECTED WRITINGS, pp, 15-16

†Barnard 2002, pp 140-1. From this point in the book, the Twelve Great Remedies will be referred to as the Twelve Healers.

comprised collectives, or groups, and that each of us belongs to one of these 'soul groups'. His message in all of this was that our own spiritual responsibility, along with that of our soul companions, is about transformation.

By working through the hindrance or soul lesson of our particular soul collective we have the opportunity to realize its 'virtue'. Thus, by engaging in the process of our soul's lesson, we each carry out our responsibility of imparting its particular virtue to the rest of humanity.* For every one of us, this is our service for all humankind, which is brotherhood in the widest sense. In our soul-work, the Twelve Healers themselves are agents of connection and change, for they shift the place of our consciousness from inward absorption to outward awareness. Further, in our 'work', we can think of the soul hindrances identified by Bach as negative soul states and conversely the virtues as positive soul states. This exemplar is in perfect harmony with the universe from the perspective of both science and spirit. In all of nature, science works in polarities and in parallels and so does the spiritual plane:

> *We would draw your attention to the importance of balance. These two aspects, light and dark, positive and negative, are working together to bring about balance and equilibrium, which is one of the fundamental laws of life. The ultimate is absolute balance within the microcosm, and within the macrocosm.†*

Our development of awareness brings us to discover that compromised emotions can lead us into a place of self-absorption and illusion. In this space it's impossible for us to offer service, much less take on this responsibility in the spirit of brotherhood. From this perspective Bach be-

*Barnard, 2002, p. 139
†White Eagle, ON THE GREAT SPIRIT, p. 46

lieved that if we can identify our soul lesson (through the soul profiles of his Twelve Healers) we have the opportunity for transformation. And, once we make this discovery, we're better able to move forward on our evolutionary path.

While Bach has a great deal to say on this subject, it's important for us to keep in mind, and appreciate, that he himself was on a journey of continual soul growth and awareness. As a true mystic and healer, he had the ability to facilitate the connection between his mind and intuitive heart, but this doesn't mean his path was clear or easy. As his understanding and intuitive abilities deepened, he made modifications in some details and impressions concerning the remedies as a system of healing.

While there are slight variances in his philosophical language depending on the audience he was addressing and his own level of awareness, the essential spirit of his message remains constant. At their foundation, the Twelve Healers are soul medicine, capable of shining light into the hidden corners of one's soul. They provide a bridge of light between the soul and our conscious awareness, bringing the wisdom held safely within the intuitive heart upwards into our conscious reality. In SOME FUNDAMENTAL CONSIDERATIONS OF DISEASE AND CURE, Bach refers to the highest class of plants and their healing qualities as having 'the power to elevate our vibrations, and thus draw down spiritual power, which cleanses mind and body, and heals'.* However, he also recognized there was more involved in removing illness and disease than each being able to identify their soul lesson. He concluded we exhibit 'mood states' and chronic personality characteristics on the mundane level as well. In this awareness, he recognized that mood states and personality characteristics could prevent the discovery of our

*Barnard, COLLECTED WRITINGS, p. 161

soul type. Additionally, he maintained that these states and characteristics directly affected our state of health. Thus, the successful treatment of illness depends upon identifying these. He believed that negative moods and personality characteristics could be so entrenched within us that until these were addressed and brought into a state of balance, one could not possibly identify the soul type and its lesson with any accuracy.*

Bach first wrote of this realization in THE TWELVE HEALERS AND FOUR HELPERS. In this book, he further describes the four additional remedies he thought of as adjuncts or helpers. These later evolved into a group of seven to complete the first nineteen of the thirty-eight Bach remedies. However, throughout his work, Bach maintained that our foundation is anchored in our soul type and the lesson meant for us to learn and teach.

To Bach's way of thinking, there was always something new to learn, or something upon which to expand. As an example, there is a variance in the language he used in FREE THYSELF. In it Bach maintains 'there is no failure when you are doing your utmost, whatever the apparent result'.† Conversely, he uses the term 'failing' and 'spiritual failings' in both his early descriptions of the first twelve remedies and in his later writings. Besides these descriptions, he seems to have also used the words, 'qualities to develop' 'weakness' and 'soul lessons' interchangeably in his writings. Through what Barnard identifies as 'the architecture of the twelve healers',§ Bach laid out the pattern of both the spiritual failings (hindrances, weakness) and corresponding virtues (soul lessons, qualities to develop) as they correspond to the

---

*The issues of mood states and personality types will be addressed in succeeding chapters.

†Barnard, COLLECTED WRITINGS, p. 70.   §ibid., p. 107

remedies known as the Twelve Healers in the context of soul types:

Failing	Herb (Soul Type)	Virtue
Fear	Mimulus	Sympathy
Weakness	Centaury	Strength
Doubt	Gentian	Understanding
Indecision	Scleranthus	Steadfastness
Ignorance	Cerato	Wisdom
Grief	Water Violet	Joy
Restraint	Chicory	Love
Indifference	Clematis	Gentleness
Terror	Rock Rose	Courage
Restlessness	Agrimony	Peace
Over-enthusiasm	Vervain	Tolerance
Impatience	Impatiens	Forgiveness

Clearly, each of Bach's soul types also can reflect temporary emotional states or characteristics of the personality. Leaving this acknowledgment aside, his concept of soul types implies that a karmic soul lesson is involved for each type, and that in these lessons, there's an emphasis on the need for a transformation. Such transformations involve the complexities of expansion in their height and depth of understanding.

SEVEN

—

As Above, so Below: Transforming
Soul lessons of Heaven and Earth

AMERICAN physician and author, Charles Glass-
man, reminds us that 'When we hold onto worry,
regret and anger, peace of mind, strength of body
and freedom of spirit eludes us.' Truer words were never
spoken. As we travel along our evolutionary pilgrimage, it's
vital for each of us to comprehend that we're spirit in body
first, but at the same time, we're compelled to walk our path
in the temporal realm. In order to manifest our soul's vision
and evolution when we hold onto negative emotions, at the
very least, we're setting ourselves up for disappointment.

On our evolutionary journey, our ego can become demanding and misguided, tightening the grip on unrealistic expectations. This is not new news. Dr Bach in his time
warned us of such negativity, including greed, bitterness,
resentment, fear and a host of other toxic emotions. As a
result, these emotions that keep us from soul growth have
no place in the realm of the higher mind. On our path,
we need to remember that this elevated realm is a link to
the pure wisdom of our soul through our heart-based intuition. By facilitating a release of the ego's idealistic fantasies,
Bach's remedies can move us forward on the journey the
universe intends for each of us.

This release is crucial if we're to make progress in embracing and manifesting the Aquarian consciousness of

global unity. In this, Bach's concept of the twelve soul types (or soul personalities) and their corresponding lessons becomes a significant consideration in the pursuit of discovering our evolutionary path. To Bach's way of thinking, our soul type is our foundation, much like the operating system is with a computer. As each of us comes into this life with our particular type, we carry a sacred lesson meant to strengthen us – as we saw in the previous chapter. Thus, when we incarnate in this lifetime, our soul is in some degree of 'contraction' or weakness with a mandate to work toward 'expansion' or strength through its lesson.

While we may manifest bits and pieces of various soul types as we evolve through an incarnation, Bach maintained that ultimately each of us remains bonded to one distinct type represented by one of the Twelve Healers. And this, in fact, remains our foundation in each lifetime.* From a spiritual perspective, it appears Bach believed we work our way through each of the twelve types and their lessons as we cycle through successive reincarnations---not unlike the philosophy found in the western system of Evolutionary Astrology. In working with its intended lesson in each life, the soul strengthens the qualities of its particular type by gleaning experience and knowledge as it moves closer to the Divine.

As Bach's work evolved, an additional twenty-six remedies became part of his repertoire. The work on these was done between 1933 and 1935, at which point he announced his work complete. Since his death in 1936, there have been those proposing that several of the additional twenty-six are also 'soul type' remedies. However, Bach mentions none of these additional remedies in the context of 'soul type' remedies; and so it would appear that in his mind, they were

*Barnard, 2002, p. 283

not. From the *spiritual* perspective, it's important to remember that Bach believed the first set of remedies, the Twelve Healers, were meant to assist the corresponding soul types in the transformation of their karmic lessons.

However, for now we need to turn from spiritual matters to an examination of the Twelve Healers, a selection of the additional twenty-six remedies and their relationship to the healing process on the mundane level. On this level, the Twelve Healers and the twenty-six additional remedies function similarly to the concept of 'root and branch herbs' used in oriental medicine or 'constitutional and lower potency' remedies used in homeopathy. In these medical traditions (and in Edward Bach's philosophy), there is always an underlying 'root' cause for a chronic imbalance, but this cause is not always in evidence. In Chinese medicine, the particular herb (or herbs) used to address the root imbalance is considered the 'principal herb'; and in homeopathy, practitioners look to identify the 'constitutional type' of the patient and its corresponding remedy. But before these solutions become clear, other support-herbs or homeopathic remedies of various potencies may be needed to help balance out the overlaying symptoms. Thus, by the clearing away of these symptoms, the imbalance at the 'root of the matter' can then be recognized and addressed. Bach practitioners refer to this process as a 'peeling of the onion'. If one reads Bach's own words carefully in THE TWELVE HEALERS AND FOUR HELPERS, published by C. W. Daniel Co. in 1933, he clearly lays out his philosophy on this issue as it relates to this concept with the flower remedies:

> *It will be found that certain cases do not seem to fit exactly any one of the Twelve Healers, and many of these are such as those who have become so used to disease that it appears to be part of their*

nature; and it is difficult to see their true selves because, instead of seeking a cure, they have adapted themselves and altered their lives to suit the disease.... Such people have lost much of their individuality, of their personality, and need to be helped out of the rut, out of the groove, in which they have become fixed before it is possible to know which of the twelve healers they need ... and the Four Helpers get us over this stage and bring us into the range of the Twelve Healers. Of course, in all healing there must be a desire in the patient to get well. *

So, while it may seem that some additional remedies discovered after the Twelve Healers might also be identified as 'soul types', this appears not to be the case in Bach's mind. Instead, as Bach stressed, there can be emotional issues that are chronic, so much so that the person is emotionally 'stuck'. In these circumstances, the remedy or remedies called for may *appear* as soul type remedies, but while the Twelve Healers can be applied to temporary or chronic emotional states, at the end of the day, the remaining twenty-six are not meant to be identified as soul types.

On our journey, we may need to call upon several of the additional twenty-six remedies; but in doing so, it's important that we maintain efforts toward the identification of our core. Although we may not be able to identify this with certainty, there's still great value in this effort. In it rests the understanding of the obstacles that keep us from moving forward both spiritually and temporally. With the help of the Twelve Healers, this is our starting point: a place from which we can steadily work to develop the characteristics of our soul's strength. Working with intent, we can move forward.

Along with the complex patterns of emotions and feel-

*Barnard, COLLECTED WRITINGS, p.70

ings that we saw when meeting our elemental dragons, each of Bach's twelve soul types also exhibit metaphorical characteristics of fire, earth, air and water. As was mentioned in earlier chapters, the purpose found in the spiritual law of reincarnation is to give our soul opportunity for growth toward perfection through the vehicle of the body and its emotions. This perpetual expedition is often referred to in spiritual teachings as the 'baptism of the four elements'. With each incarnation, our soul has the opportunity of gathering maturity through the lessons of its type. In addition, these teachings also inform us that steady growth does not always happen in each lifetime. For example, there are incarnations in which we might remain stagnantly attached to our weaknesses or failings. When this happens, we're too earthbound, ungrounded, adrift or on fire. These emotional states can be so intense or entrenched that we have little chance of connecting to our mystical path or *finding the story in our soul*.

The question then becomes, how do we identify our soul type? While it's not impossible to identify, there's no quick solution, simply because by nature we're challenged to take an objective inventory of our behaviour or ourselves. Still, we have clues at our disposal from both our external and internal environments if we pay attention. These clues, however, can come cloaked in a myriad of configurations including our natal Moon, which we shall soon see.

Psychological theory suggests we're mirrors for each other – the habits and conduct that we find offensive in others may in fact be characteristic of our own nature, signalling that we need to take a closer look at ourselves. Other clues may reside in difficult relationships and/or careers that we've consciously but misguidedly chosen. Chronic physical illnesses or accidents also give us opportunities to examine ourselves in depth. Such clues heading the pack of likely suspects inform us that familiar habits and/or responses are now no longer viable if we wish to move forward in our evolution.

So once again our process and progress depends upon our willingness to examine what it is in us that's keeping us 'stuck'. If we take a pass on this commitment, we end up recreating the same script over and over, but with different casts of characters. Once we're able to make a list of possibilities for change, we're then able to survey the characteristics of the Twelve Healers not only as remedies to call upon, but as soul type candidates so that we may get on with our work.

Recalling Bach's philosophy relating to the healing action of the remedies, it's important to remember that it's the positive energy or life force of each remedy that shifts the negative characteristics of the particular soul type, bringing it into the brilliance of its intended expansion. In this, from the spiritual perspective, we have the opportunity to meet the core of the Twelve Healers and the light they bring into obscured aspects of our soul. And now, it's time to inspect the negative and positive states for each of them.

EIGHT

———

The Twelve Great Remedies

*Healing is to give a person the skills to see the miracle of
their own existence and that of a flower's. And, even further,
how the two are connected.*

Shawn May, American Writer

S EEMINGLY the ever-present and optimistic diplomat,
avoiding all confrontation, the ***Agrimony*** soul appears
as the peacemaker who is very much 'out there' with
boundless energy actively connected in and to the world.
However, there's only one slight problem… what the rest of
the world is seeing is the negative Agrimony soul type, and as
such, it's the master of disguise. In this state, the Agrimony
soul fools the world. This type appears to others as *the one who
'has it together'* but the reality is that its weakness is its *restlessness*
at the soul level. Behind every smile, every laugh, this soul
struggles with its disquiet in silent torment no one else ever
sees. Simply put, Agrimony can't find the peace that is its lesson and strength. Without question, the worst thing for this
constricted soul is that its secret torment will be revealed and
that it will be exposed. In order to cope, it will, often unconsciously, hide its distress by retreating to the use of drugs, alcohol, or other addictive behaviours. This method of retreat
or 'protection' of course only creates more difficulties.

It's almost as if, in this state, the Agrimony soul is in the
wrong incarnation, the wrong body, trying unsuccessfully to

throw these things off, like too many covers on the bed. From the spiritual perspective, they are in the right body and in the right place at the right time. The challenge for the Agrimony soul is to become comfortable revealing who and particularly how they really are. Nevertheless, in the negative state, these individuals will reply that they are 'just fine' when asked; never mind they have just filed for bankruptcy, their partner has left them, and that government revenue agents have them on their 'most-wanted list' for tax misunderstandings. Agrimony as a remedy assists these souls in developing the ability to be verbally honest about their state of being. Once they work with this challenge, they find that their restlessness dissipates – and in their liberation, they can move forward on their journey in a soulful quality of *peace*. In writing about the lesson of peace for Agrimony, Bach said:

> *Does not Agrimony open the door to let in the golden vital breath of peace instead of love? One always feels that the light of Agrimony is so very closely associated with 'the peace that passeth understanding', the peace of the Christ.*

Although peace is the specific soul lesson for Agrimony, Bach also made it a repetitive theme, woven in throughout his philosophy. In his address, 'Ye Suffer From Yourselves', he identifies the state of peace as being one of the basic components required for healing. Bach 'saw' that a hospital of the future would be:

> *A sanctuary of peace, hope and joy. No hurry; no noise: entirely devoid of all the terrifying apparatus and appliances of today.... The object of all institutions will be to have an atmosphere of peace, and of hope, of joy, and of faith.* *

If you're launching a new enterprise requiring collec-

*Barnard, COLLECTED WRITINGS, p. 115

tive participation, particularly an effort that focuses upon fighting for justice, get an 'expanded' **Vervain** soul on your steering committee – if you can find one. More than likely, however, you'll be confronted by the over-zealous enthusiasm of a negative Vervain soul on a mission. In this state, these soul types can be extremely difficult to work with. Unlike compromised Agrimony, who struggles with his or her personal experience of microcosm versus macrocosm, negative Vervain simply is dissatisfied with the entire macrocosmic set-up. In the contracted extreme, the Vervain souls are frothing at the mouth, determined. They'll do everything possible to get their oar into the water, paddling furiously to engineer the tides of change – for the betterment of humankind, of course, or their next-door neighbour.

Among the Twelve Healers, Bach identified Vervain as the 'enthusiast'. In the negative state, the Vervain soul suffers from an overabundance of a driving force whose weakness or hindrance is one of *over-enthusiasm*. Emotional fire of this nature translates into intolerance of others and ideas that don't match Vervain's own. Because these souls have travelled far on their journey, they have developed an indomitable spirit and bring with them very clear ideals of 'how things should be'. The problem is not in the intent, but in the application. In this state the Vervain soul hits the ground running, taking no prisoners.

Those whom we experience in this way may or may not be actual Vervain types. However, if they are, it's quite possible they've karmically chosen to be in relationships that exhibit similar behaviour either through demand for notable achievement, critical role-models, or both. This being the case, the Vervain soul has the option of remaining stagnant by mimicking these behaviours and philosophies or embracing its soul-remedy to assist it as it learns the lesson of *tolerance*. Bach identified Vervain's potential power as that seen in leaders and effective teachers. Should contracted Vervain souls take the option of learning tolerance, they can embrace this power through the spiritual axiom that all great work can be accomplished quietly.

While poor Centaury struggles to learn about setting boundaries (as we shall soon see) in the negative state, the fiery **Impatiens** soul knows exactly where the boundaries are and wants to burn them down; the sooner, the better. In its very nature, negative Impatiens is a bundle of combustible energy in thought and action. This type is blessed with a quicksilver mind, but when it gets entrenched in its failing of *impatience*, it perceives everything and everyone around it as unnecessary and irrelevant restrictions.

In other words, 'get out of my way' is its message to the world and Impatiens manifests this by striking out through caustic verbiage and visible irritation. If this soul does not move forward in learning its lesson of *forgiveness*, it finds that it's alienated those around it and a destiny of leading a lifetime filled with loneliness. In the learning of its lesson of forgiveness, the challenge for Impatiens souls is to recognize that not everyone thinks like, or as fast, as they. A major key to attaining progress on their path is by working with their soul-remedy, Impatiens. This remedy helps to bring this soul to an awareness that others have gifts to offer and further, that we're all connected through our contributions and universal brotherhood.

As with each of the soul types, it's impossible for us to know why someone comes into this incarnation with a particular soul lesson to learn instead of another. Barnard and others confidently identify Bach as an Impatiens type,* It's interesting to note that in sketching a verbal profile of Bach,

*For example, Barnard, 2002, p. 32

his close colleague, Dr. F. J. Wheeler, notes that:

> *His intense desire to help others to understand and learn as quickly as he did himself sometimes made him impatient at slowness, but this mood would not last long [author note: Impatiens characteristics]... although he was quick to anger at injustice, unhesitatingly voicing it and siding with the weaker [author note: Vervain characteristics], he would encourage the weak one to fight his own battles and so regain his self-esteem.* *

It may be that Bach himself was an example of someone whose overlying characteristics are so strong that it is tricky to identify the soul type. Thus, perhaps to the world Bach appeared as an Impatiens type when actually he was a Vervain soul, clearly on a karmic mission for this lifetime. Bach may have been one of those people with whom the personality characteristics (Impatiens) were so entrenched that they hid the actual soul type (Vervain). What is paramount to remember, however, is that the remedies can bring unique awareness, lessons, and experience to each of us in our efforts to identify and work our intended soul lesson for this lifetime.

The negative state of the soul type **Mimulus**, is about *fear* – fear that specifically possesses earthbound or worldly characteristics. Fear of the dark, fear of flying, fear of mice ... phobias of worldly things we can name. As a soul type, the contracted state of Mimulus manifests as visceral fear felt within our very core and, as an unbridled feeling, it's emotionally toxic. Bach described Mimulus soul types as being quietly afraid both of things they can name and/or of things that might never happen. From this perspective, Mimulus types are always 'on guard' against what in the extreme is *anything and everything with a worldly name attached to it.*

The remedy, Mimulus, engages the intellect to overcome

*Barnard, 2002, p. 112

these fears, giving it the ability to sort through the reality rationally. This then gives the person the ability to stand firm in the face of challenges. With the help of this remedy, these types can work toward their soul-mission, which is to teach the virtue or quality of *sympathy* for others because they can well understand their quiet desperation.

While negative states of feeling can lead some souls to become self-absorbed, they can also fluctuate the other way and become what psychologists often label as being co-dependent. Co-dependency is a personality characteristic where the negative state of the **Centaury** soul lives. With a misaligned earthly passion and desire to serve, Centaury's hindrance or *weakness* is the inability or lack of will to set boundaries by saying: 'No'.

As a result, one can become the common doormat by default, doing too much for others while sacrificing its own well-being from a severely skewed altruistic perspective. As with all contracted or negative states of feeling, this perspective comes with its own set of difficulties. Foremost among these difficulties is the danger of unknowingly engineering one's fate toward becoming a sacrificial lamb, physically and emotionally. With the inability to set boundaries against the demands of others, there's a drive to continually 'do' for them while the Centaury's physical and emotional resources slowly go down the drain. Because these types have sacrificed and lost their will, it's only when they're 'on the ropes' that they may wonder, if at all, how they arrived at such a state.

Another difficulty with the vulnerable Centaury soul is that of the well-intended but misguided desire to 'fix' problems others are experiencing. Within the law of karma, our soul sets up difficult relationships and/or situations meant to offer us opportunities for paying back karmic debt in return for soul growth. However, when we interfere with others' affairs by attempting to fix their problems, this effort actually stalls *their* evolutionary process. As a result, the motivational experience of distress required for another's transformation is delayed or altogether derailed.

Here again, we see the inability to set personal boundaries as a major challenge to this aspect of Centaury. Those who incarnate with a Centaury soul and its lesson are natural servers, but the lack of balance creates the inability to stay focused on 'their own side of the street'. This behaviour delays the soul's evolution because of the inability of shifting towards the expanded state or virtue of *strength of will*. Edward Bach believed that when Centaury types have learned their soul lesson, with the help of the Centaury remedy, they will have come 'a very long way along the road to being of great service once [they have realized] that [they] must be a little more positive in [their] live[s]'.*

For most of us, the experience of self-doubt and its companion, a feeling of failure, are natural emotions – part and parcel of the human incarnation. For **Gentian** soul types, however, *self-doubt* is a destructive weakness. In the negative soul-state, these individuals begin with a positive passion for their direction in life and the tasks required to reach their goals. However, when difficulty emerges at the first bend in the road, when an obstacle, no matter how minor, appears, discouragement and self-doubt readily take hold. At this juncture, Gentian soul types who have not progressed in mastering the expanded emotional state of this remedy become easily discouraged, ready to throw in the towel and give up. Recalling Bach's philosophy on failure, his message was specifically directed to these soul types with the *understanding that there is no failure when you are doing your utmost, whatever the apparent result*.†

*Barnard, 2002, p. 112   †Barnard, COLLECTED WRITINGS, p. 161

The challenge, then, for Gentian souls is to embrace the virtue of understanding. In order to connect to its soul's intended evolutionary purpose, the Gentian type needs to understand that steady perseverance is essential to overcoming self-doubt. While faith in self is important for each of the soul types, it's particularly important for this type. For them, a vital key is to remember that cosmic law dictates trusting the perfect timing of the universe; that the universe provides us with whatever we need for our expansion and growth. For the soul type who finds change and challenge difficult, Gentian helps them to understand the value of, and engage in, perseverance in the face of adversity and disappointment.

Listening to the wisdom and truth of its own heart and being able to *speak* it is the challenge for a **Cerato** soul. The irony of this soul type is that it's highly intuitive, but because of the weakened state, it dwells in *ignorance* or *foolishness*, unable to recognize its strength rests in its own *wisdom*. Lacking in the ability to find its voice, these souls don't have a clue who they are or what they need to do. The weak Cerato soul is not so much one who experiences stolen identity, but one with a case of *lost* identity. Having no faith in its own judgment, this soul type perceives its intuitive, authentic voice as something suspect. Chronically seeking direction from others, they have great difficulty in accessing their higher self and its wisdom and thus have great trouble in finding their intended path.

Another aspect to Cerato souls is that they always want to do the right thing. In this desire, they feed upon the misguided notion that the more information they have, the better off they are in their quest. Unfortunately, this chronic 'gathering' of information from others does nothing other than result in stagnation. Because this Cerato soul can't hear, much less listen to its intuitive wisdom in all of its 'gathering', it can never act upon anything with conviction. Vacillation, making foolish decisions and taking foolish actions does nothing but further detain its progress. Unable to hold on to a decision, along with dependence upon guidance from others, creates an appearance of being ungrounded and 'ignorant', one of the very words Bach used to describe the failing of Cerato subjects.

In HEAL THYSELF, Bach notes that, when ill, Cerato types 'try any and every cure suggested'.* It may be that it's the unrealized types who, in their desperation to learn and do the right thing, lead the pack of the 'sacred shoppers'. In working with the Cerato remedy, Bach maintained that this soul type could be 'freed from outside influences, [enabling them] to use the great gift of wisdom [they] possess for the good of mankind'.† However, for the contracted Cerato soul, the quality of trusting its intuitive voice and speaking it to guide others lies dormant. At the end of the day, it functions in the world as a follower, deaf to its intended virtue of wisdom.

Another soul type that in its negative state struggles with deciding is the **Scleranthus** type. However, unlike the Cerato soul who has an identity crisis, Scleranthus types know who they are, but all things being equal, can't decide whether they should wear the black dress or the white dress to the ball, buy the Mini Cooper or the Bentley. While the Cerato soul runs around asking everyone what they should do, the Scleranthus soul relies on its intellect while considering its choices. As a result, this individual directs all of its energy to the head and thus can't verbalize easily. Being unable to have their cake and eat it too results in quiet distress that manifests in first deciding one thing and then another, because all the options and possibilities are attractive. Being

*Barnard, COLLECTED WRITINGS, p. 84   †ibid., p. 108

mental or too much in the head, the contracted Scleranthus soul lacks the ability to access its intuition. Unable to settle on anything requires a tremendous expenditure of energy, draining the person to the point of powerlessness.

In SOME FUNDAMENTAL CONSIDERATIONS OF DISEASES AND CURE, Bach initially called Scleranthus types 'weathervanes', which is an accurate reflection of their inconsistent decision-making skills.* At first glance, such patterns seem identical to those of the vulnerable Cerato soul. However, in describing the hindrances of the Scleranthus soul, Bach focused on the mental aspect, observing that this type suffers from mental torment. These soul types process their dilemmas mentally while Cerato has to verbalize its process – two unique ways of being – but neither type can plug into its intuition. Scleranthus' virtue and strength lie in acquiring the ability to remain steadfast in its decisions. Similar to Cerato's soul-issue, the challenge for the contracted Scleranthus soul is to find comfort in trusting its intuition and letting it be the guide in the decision-making process. Letting the intuitive heart guide the head, not the other way round, is the key for the Scleranthus type in discovering its soul's purpose and path.

The Water Violet plant, according to Julian Barnard, is an ancient one with a complex history that mirrors the characteristics of the **Water Violet** soul type.† In spiritual teachings, those who are considered 'old souls' come into this incarnation possessing a vast storehouse of experience and wisdom; these are the fruits of their labours through many lifetimes. However, the hindrance of the Water-Violet soul is that its history, both karmic and present, has produced a state of *grief*. As is true for each of us, the cosmic

*Barnard, COLLECTED WRITINGS, p. 168
†Barnard, 2002, p. 123

laws of karma and rebirth give us the experience of both joy and sorrow. But, for the Water-Violet soul, a facet of their sorrow or grief stems from repeated experiences of betrayal. In their silent grief, negative Water Violet comes off as keeping 'a stiff upper lip', while appearing detached, prideful, and aloof. Realistically, this behaviour is a means of emotional protection. Even in simple friendship, intimacy is a hardship. Even more of a challenge is finding a level of comfort in the intimacy of a romantic relationship. Physically, the contracted emotional state of this soul type makes its subjects appear rigid and apart from others, as they exude an air of superiority and entitlement.

Water-violet souls have the lesson of this lifetime of learning the virtue of *joy* by sharing their wisdom of experience through participation in the environment surrounding them. In working through emotional excavation using Water Violet as a remedy, the resulting connection to their feelings brings an awareness that detachment is the source of their grief and, what was once good for them – an old defense mechanism that worked – is no longer serving them well. When this happens, the emotional armour begins to disintegrate, and they skillfully learn to balance the need for personal space and the extension of brotherhood through service.

Having explored metaphors for the emotions of fire, earth and air, we now come to the emotions of the last element, that of water. Esoteric tradition teaches that water is the metaphor for feelings and emotions, but among the Twelve Healers, the three soul types of **Chicory, Clematis and Rock Rose** particularly reflect sensitivity to emotions and feelings identified with this element.

The **Chicory** soul loves to love; but in its negative state, this soul can become tenacious, self-absorbed, and controlling. As a plant, Chicory adapts to its surrounding environment, manifesting characteristics of changeability in order to fit the situation. This is perhaps why Bach wrote several different descriptions of the negative Chicory soul type as the repertoire evolved. He was exceptionally critical of this soul-state in his early paper, *Some Fundamental Considerations on Disease and Cure*, written in 1930. Here he identified Chicory souls as egotistical, spiteful, revengeful and cruel depending on the situation. He later softened his description, settling for the word *'restraint'* in describing this type's weakness. While restraint would seem to indicate a soul lesson rather than its weakness, this is not, apparently, what Bach saw.

Instead, he identified Chicory's weakness as *unable to restrain itself* through emotional manipulation. By instigating feelings of guilt (family is a particularly popular target), the contracted Chicory soul type can go to extremes, contriving situations to keep targets close. Using narcissistic strategies, they succeed in their goal of getting their own way. In many respects, the immature Chicory soul is very needy at a deep level, probably because this soul has experienced similar parenting dynamics during its own history. Of course, as with each of the soul types, such characteristics can manifest in infancy and the soul type is no different. Indications of this state in a Chicory infant may surface as constant demands to be held and/or nursed. As the infant grows, the child can show up as an obstreperous little horror. The danger here is that those whom the Chicory soul is attempting to control may eventually rebel dramatically in order to gain their freedom. This is especially true with a parent who manipulates his or her children under the guise of 'knowing what's best for them', only to lose their love.

Bach described the strength of this soul type as *love;*

making the point that we gain love by giving others freedom without expectation. In working with the Chicory remedy, subjects of this soul type mature by finding that by giving freedom rather than holding on, they gain a far deeper and more global love than they ever thought possible.

Coming to the feelings and weakness of the *Clematis* soul, we find *indifference* which shows up by appearing ungrounded and dreamy. In *Some Fundamental Considerations of Disease and Cure*, Bach originally described the Clematis soul as 'the ecstatic'.* Recalling from Chapter Four that we are all 'called to be mystics', we may appreciate that characteristics of ecstasy – such as 'bliss' or 'rapture', identified with some 'mystics' – are not necessarily a prerequisite for mysticism. In other words, not all mystics are ecstatics or Clematis souls.

However, when identifying the 'hindrance state' of this soul type, Bach was referring to those souls who chronically prefer to escape into the realms of their ideals and visions with little concern for, or fear of, illness or death. As a defense mechanism, and to protect their highly sensitive natures like the crab, they retreat into their shell when faced with problems or hard realities. For the negative Clematis soul, living in the reality of the present seems too harsh and overwhelming; it's as if they can't muster the internal strength to interact with even the very ordinary details of life. Thus, their heightened sensitivity to the energy and emotional states of others and their own surrounding environment makes this method of escape their modus operandi; they simply aren't present. This state of non-presence can manifest in a varied assortment of both physical and mental behaviours. Vulnerable states of the Clematis soul can range from daydreaming, fainting, or Attention Deficit

*Barnard, COLLECTED WRITINGS, p. 165

Disorder to the extreme of dementia or Alzheimer's disease.

The virtue or strength of the Clematis soul is one of *gentleness*, but it's a virtue that can only be realized with stability and a sense of being grounded into the earth through its soul-remedy. The Clematis remedy assists these souls in becoming earthbound, supporting them in ways that help them respond self-assuredly with gentleness, rather than retreating in escape. With their sensitivity to others and the world around them, these soul types have the opportunity and responsibility to teach the rest of the world the value of extending gentleness to each other … a virtue sorely needed in today's world and an absolute necessity for spreading global brotherhood.

As with the water signs in astrology, heightened sensitivity is a double-edged sword. For the **Rock Rose** soul, this sensitivity is more amplified than in either Chicory or Clematis souls. At the cellular level, there's an awareness of vulnerability that conveys a palpable terror. Just the 'business of being' is terrifying; and thus *terror* is the weakness or hindrance for these souls. For them, this weakness manifests in a constant emotional undercurrent of belief about 'not coming through it', whatever 'it' is. Interestingly, this undercurrent can remain well-hidden until that time when it bursts up and out, manifesting into a full-blown, paralysing panic attack. Unlike the visible timidity and nervousness of the Mimulus soul, the hidden terror for Rock Rose is really only recognizable to those who possess similar soul characteristics. It's very difficult for a non-Rock Rose soul to detect this in others because of Rock Rose's remarkable ability to 'stuff it'. In reality, the accurate identification of this soul type only becomes a conscious consideration when its negative characteristics visibly manifest in chronic episodes of panic and terror.

From a karmic perspective, the contracted soul-state of Rock Rose isn't something that has just come about in this lifetime. More than likely, this state of contraction results from many lifetimes in which they have experienced the 'fires of hell', so to speak, and consequently paralysing terror has become a thematic state of being. Bach identified these souls as being terrified of things other than the material, such as death, suicide, or the supernatural. According to him, with the help of its soul-remedy, the lesson or positive quality for the Rock Rose soul is to develop courage in this lifetime. As these souls learn to become comfortable with the emotional state of courage, they begin to expand and can progressively stand firm in their place. With new-found courage, they're further able to displace the contracted emotional shadow of terror that has made their lives difficult and fraught with unrealized contributions to humanity. In coming to grips with this debilitating emotion, they can then teach others that we are divinely protected and that therefore, terror is only a shadow.

As healing tools, The Twelve Healers can meet us where we are; and if we are willing to follow, they can take us where our soul wants us to be – and yet, on our journey, we have more at our disposal. As I indicated earlier, uncertainty of the astrological scheme was the reason Bach dropped public mention of connection between the remedies and astrology. However, knowing he held an interest in astrology continues to fascinate and therefore justifies a closer look as it relates to our soul's evolution – which is where we're now headed.

NINE

—

The Karmic Moon: the Heart of our Story

*Healing is the domain of the Moon and perhaps
its most elemental function*

Steven Forrest

IN THE PREVIOUS chapters we explored Bach's work and his concept of soul types and/or personality types – related, as he believed, to his original Twelve Healers and his personal interest in astrology. By his own admission, there's always room for further exploration, expansion and adjustment, which is certainly the case whenever we're delving into esoteric subjects. Because he believed astrology provided a channel for discovering the soul's personality and its intended lessons, we also know of his philosophy that each zodiacal sign and chart placement of one's natal Moon is linked to one of his Twelve Healers:

> *[One's type] of personality [is] indicated to us by the Moon according to which sign of the Zodiac she is in at birth, and a study of this will give us the following points: 1. The type of personality, 2. His [her] object and his [her] work in life, [and] 3. The remedy which will assist him [her] in that work....*

> *Our personality we learn from the position of the Moon at birth; our dangers of interference from the planets.... If we can hold our personality, be true unto ourselves, we need fear no planetary or outside influence. The remedies assist us to maintain our personality.* *

*Barnard, COLLECTED WRITINGS, pp 77-8

What's interesting here is that Bach's belief in the connection between one's natal Moon and one's soul path wasn't far off from the emergence of a specialized form of western astrology roughly forty years after his death. Even so, Bach became concerned that those who had no interest in or weren't sympathetic to astrological philosophy would disregard the healing benefits of the remedies. By all indications, to address this he ceased public reference to the relationship between the two systems. It's doubtful, however, being the student of the esoteric he was, that he dropped his personal interest in astrology. In a letter written to friends while he was living in Cromer in the autumn of 1933, Bach states:

I am being very cautious as regards astrology, and that is why one left out the Signs and the months in the first Twelve Healers. This work is decidedly going to assist vastly in the purification and understanding of astrology, but my part seems to be to give general principles whereby people like you, who have a more detailed knowledge, may discover a great truth. That is why I do not wish to be associated with anything dogmatic until one is sure.*

Although in the end he left this connection aside publicly, I've always thought that privately he never lost confidence in the integration of astrology and his Twelve Healers. Still, things were changing astrologically in Bach's time and have continued to change rapidly since his death.

While Bach's brief statements on astrology focused on the Moon, with a suggestion that we need not worry about influences from the other planets, western astrology considers every placement in a chart. Symbols are the language of the universe and as such our chart holds thousands of possibilities, resulting in a web of complexities, contradictions and confusion woven against the backdrop of the universe.

*ORIGINAL WRITINGS, ed. Howard and Ramsell, p. 87

Even so, we come into this life with a chart that's perfect for us and our soul's evolution. Engaging in this process is a lifetime's worth of work as our soul offers challenging opportunities amid new astronomical and astrological revelations.

As an example, just six short years prior to Bach's death in 1936, the planet Pluto was discovered – adding yet another element for chart interpretation by astrologers. Since his death eighty-five years ago, western astrology has grown by leaps and bounds. In 1977 the asteroid, Chiron,* named for the wounded healer in mythology, was discovered, which in recent years has led to an explosion of interest in how various asteroids affect the energy in a chart. As we make new cosmic discoveries against this backdrop, what we've been witnessing since Bach's time is a morphing and expansion of western astrology into a myriad of specialities, such as Financial, Medical and Synastry Astrology and Astrocartography, just to name a few.

Among these specialities we find Evolutionary Astrology, a term first coined by Raymond Merriman, a well-known American astrologer and financial analyst in his 1977 limited edition book, EVOLUTIONARY ASTROLOGY. Less than ten years later, astrologer Jeffrey Wolf Green released PLUTO: THE EVOLUTIONARY JOURNEY OF THE SOUL (1985) followed by the first of many works on this subject produced by my teacher and mentor, Steven Forrest, beginning with his classic, THE INNER SKY (1988).

As an integrative model between astrology and holistic psychology, Evolutionary Astrology asserts that we cycle through lifetimes on our path of self-discovery and soul growth. And, despite the intent of this cyclic journey in our evolution, we need a map. This is where our astrological birth chart shines.

*To an astronomer, Chiron is properly known as a 'Centaur object'

Although our chart represents the blueprint for our soul's intended pathway this time around, the universe doesn't let us off that easily. Of course there's a catch. Through the evolutionary lens, our chart's symbols and planet placements represent the soul's condition as it incarnates into this life. With this incarnation comes a piece of emotion-based, 'unfinished karma' – what Jeffrey Wolf Green refers to as 'a skipped step'. If Bach were with us today, it's not a far stretch to imagine he would have found this perspective a fascinating complement to his own philosophy about one's life journey, that it's one in a cycle of lives through which the soul learns lessons in order to evolve.

In Evolutionary Astrology, there's the premise that we've come to a point in our process where our soul whispers that in order for us to grow, there's more emotional work that must be done. The piece of unfinished karmic business we've brought along from the past into this incarnation needs attention. The good news is that we're now courageous enough, strong enough to tackle whatever this piece represents – if we so choose to do so with the power of choice. Working with choice isn't about fate, pre-destination or voodoo. It's our soul work and we can either engage with it or not. Choices matter.

If we choose to take part using this lens of Evolutionary Astrology, the Moon in our birth chart comes to the forefront. For many reasons, as we shall see, our Moon is at the 'heart of our karmic story'. This brings us back around to Bach's placing so much importance on it from an astrological perspective and his remedies. Unfortunately, we don't have his scheme of matching lunar zodiacal signs with each of his Twelve Healers ... not one that was made public, at any rate. There may be several reasons for this. As noted, Bach was understandably cautious. His revolutionary work required integrity and credibility. We've seen by his own words that he didn't want to be dogmatic where astrology and the remedies were involved. On the other hand, it's quite possible he wasn't able to come up with a scheme with which he was satisfied.

While I recognize others may feel differently, try as I might I've not been able to match each of Bach's Twelve Healers in a way that comfortably coincides with the evolutionary intent of each Moon sign. Still, this doesn't mean we can't call upon his remedies to help us on our karmic journey, something we'll be looking at more closely shortly. But first things first, we need to start at the beginning.

Where Is Your Moon?

If you've never had an astrological reading, to answer this question you can access the graphic of your chart through a number of free internet sites, including Astrodienst (ww. astro.com). If that's the application you choose, once you're in the site:

- Click on 'Free Horoscopes' at the very top of the page
- A new page will appear. Choose 'Chart Drawing Ascendant' option under the heading for 'Horoscope Chart Drawings'

A new page will appear with an option for 'Guests'. Click on the link for data entry and follow the prompts. You'll need your date, place and time of birth (from your birth certificate*) in order to see an accurate chart.

*Note: For those born in the United States who need a copy of their birth certificate, these are usually available for a nominal fee through the County Clerk's office in the county of birth. Please also note, although unusual, not all birth certificates contain birth times depending on the country involved.

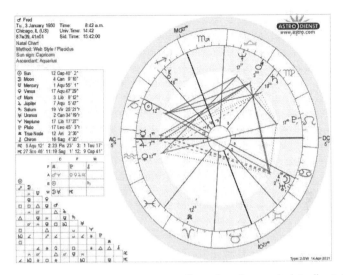

Screenshot of a sample Astrodienst chart

In the box on the left, among the list of planets you'll see the crescent symbol for the Moon right under the Sun, along with its zodiacal sign. In the chart sample pictured, the Moon is in the sign of Cancer – appearing in the lower right corner of the wheel. It's important to note here, that western astrology is based on mathematical calculations. While our Sun sign is determined by fairly consistent calendar dates, determining one's Moon sign at birth is more complicated, which is why people casually meeting up in bars aren't saying, 'I'm a Taurus Moon, what are you?'

Charts are complicated, contradictory and confusing. And in this, as our chart's luminary partner to the Sun, the Moon is incredibly critical, as Bach also believed. It represents what celebrated astrologer Noel Tyl identified as our 'reigning need'. As our soul path isn't a singular issue of conscious awareness, work takes place in the internal landscape of our 'holies of holies' where we receive important, unspoken transmissions from the Divine. It's as if this information becomes lodged deeply within us, available for access through our Moon. The Moon has no language. Its landscape is purely internal and intuitive. When we sleep, when we dream, we're ensconced in the territory of magic. At its most basic meaning, the Moon is our **heart**.

With our Moon being primal, each of its zodiacal signs has an evolutionary goal in this lifetime and a pathway toward it – or what Steven Forrest refers to as a 'strategy'. And while our unconscious, lunar process plays a big role in our evolution, there's conscious help available to us. If we're aware of the evolutionary intent of our Moon, we can use this information to help point us in the right direction as we travel along our soul's path, mis-steps and all.

Once again, it's important to remember we're talking about our 'emotional heart'. If we engage in activities that support our Moon, we feel contented, connected and at peace with the world. But when life throws us curves, when the bottom falls out, then we aren't always in such a great space, and yet we have Dr Bach's remedies to help bring us back into balance. How our emotional body responds internally to external triggers depends not only upon our Moon's sign and placement in our birth chart, but also the energy contributed by the other planets in it. Astrology is a layered business, one of the many reasons that it's a complicated system. But in the end, these factors result in a chart that's as unique for us as our fingerprint, perfect for us in this incarnation. It's ours alone – even if our best friend was born on the same day. So let's explore a little more basic astrology, as to why our astrological fingerprint is so important.

In the western system, there are twelve arenas for planet placement in a chart, otherwise known as 'houses' or 'circumstances of life'. Each one of these arenas represents a specific backdrop for 'how' the energy of the planet will behave or manifest. For example, if our Libra Moon finds its home in the mind's arena of perception and communication, the circumstances in which this Moon's emotional landscape plays out will be very different than if it were in the arena that has to do with our 'life mission' to the community at large.

With twelve zodiacal signs and twelve houses in a chart, plus influences from the other celestial bodies (including the Sun), the nuances of our Moon's reactions reach into the stratosphere – a scope far beyond this discussion. Furthermore, when considering the behaviour of the signs, there's overlap whether we're talking about the Sun, the Moon or any other planet. Each sign carries basic characteristics that never change. For example, the ego of a Gemini Sun will always be curious in its high expression, while satisfying the curiosity of its emotional heart will always feed a Gemini Moon.

While there's often a variety of possibilities and an overlap as to which of Dr Bach's remedies we may use to help balance out negative emotions, consulting his basic virtues or positive characteristics of each remedy is an excellent place to start in selecting the ones to help lift us up into a more positive emotional state. Further on, we'll be diving deeper into the karmic contract behind our Moon and taking a brief look at Bach's own chart. But first we need to take a peek at the lunar emotional signatures and evolutionary intent by sign.

TEN

—

I Would Know you Anywhere

'The sun sees your body. The Moon sees your soul'

Unknown

MOON IN ARIES ♈
In Roman mythology, Mars was the god of war, an intense guy for sure. People born with the Moon in Aries are natural defenders and protectors. The high expression of this Moon? Bring it on, sword at the ready, the ultimate competitor! But this Moon also says, if I'm not defending/protecting something, I need adventure; I need to push the envelope. Skydiving, hiking up to Machu Picchu, count me in! At the end of the day, the ultimate goal for an Aries Moon is the engagement of courage, whether it's standing up for someone unable to defend themselves, speaking truth or having an attitude of 'the torpedoes be damned'. These all require courage in the guise of pure will. As Eleanor Roosevelt said, 'Do one thing every day that scares you'.

This is the Aries Moon in her high expression. As Aries is a fire sign, these Moons can easily assume there's aggression directed toward them where none exists. Defensive emotions of rage, anger, bullying, and cruel behaviour can show their ugly faces in a heartbeat. Lashing out in knee-jerk fashion in the need to be 'right' without the brain engaged is high on the list of unattractive behaviours when

Aries goes off the rails.

For all of us, words matter, and when the emotion of fear takes over, an Aries Moon can be as damaging with words as physically abusive. Conversely, the healthy Moon thrives on winning, but the process needs to be done with heart-centered intent rather than ego-centered intent.

MOON IN TAURUS ♉

With peace-loving Taurus following Aries in the Zodiac, the war is over. For the Taurus Moon, the primary goal is to calm down and to learn to trust its intuition. A Taurus Moon isn't particularly complicated. Taurus is earthy and has an affinity to the natural world and, with this, to things and an environment that are beautiful and simple. All it really needs and wants is to feel safe and to be at peace. At its core, these things feed and nurture it.

Basic, uncomplicated things in life such as the beauty of music, art, being outside, or an intimate setting around a good meal by candlelight with family or friends delight this Moon. Taurus needs to stay grounded and to just be real in the moment. Food, water, clothing, shelter, safety – things found at the base of American psychologist Abraham Maslow's famous 'Hierarchy of Needs' – are of primal importance for a Taurus Moon.

Having the evolutionary intent of bringing the heart to a place of accepting its need for simplicity and internal peace without drama, Taurus can get tripped up by getting too attached to material 'things'. It can mistake possessions as a reflection of personal identity, values, and misguided safety. In other words, 'if I have this, this is who I am, and it keeps me safe.'

This mis-step is especially true for those who suffer from a sense of low self-esteem. Another vulnerability for a

Taurus Moon is that change is difficult. Change feels 'unsafe' and this can lead to holding onto things that no longer serve well. Spiralling into intransigence, stubbornness and rigidity, represented by the Bull, a Taurus Moon can plant her hooves into the ground for eternity. This can lead to a recycling of hard lessons through lifetimes, when the path forward is knowing what to hold on to and what to let go of in the spirit of evolutionary growth.

MOON IN GEMINI ♊

With its direct relationship to the god Mercury, 'messenger of the gods', communication and curiosity in full sway rest at the heart of this Moon's evolutionary goal. In her high expression, a Gemini Moon possesses an innate knowing that there's more out there than what she thinks she knows or sees. And because everything is all so interesting, there's no holding back in the need to discover and constantly learn if she's true to herself. Even when this Moon is experiencing her own process of death, there's a part of her that's fascinated.

The need for mental stimulation and the opportunity for change are paramount for this Moon, as well as finding her voice through the art of lively conversation. However, the sharing of ideas and exchange of information can be stalled by scattered attention. It's not so much about the information *per se*, but the process, the experience. This characteristic is so basic in Gemini, that in trying to follow its unstoppered flow of words, even the most determined Taurus Moon can become exasperated!

For Gemini, boredom is simply not an option, and the prospect of this is equal to the despair of a death knell. In addition, there's also an evolutionary obligation that requires this Moon to listen as well as well as speak.

When it trips into its low expression, the Gemini Moon retreats behind words rather than dealing with feelings too difficult to handle. Confronted by the dragons who push to dive deep where the emotional muck lurks, walls made of words suddenly appear as protection from inconvenient truths, stalling the evolution of the Gemini heart.

MOON IN CANCER ♋

Following the mental busy-ness of Gemini in the zodiac, we find Cancer, the Great Mother. Because this sign is ruled by the Moon in western astrology, individuals born with a Cancer Moon possess the gift of a natural healer and com-forter-in-chief for the rest of us, whether or not they're aware of this.

While nurturing and 'caring for' are innate to Cancer, it can easily fall into the trap of psychological co-dependen-cy, too much 'mothering' or rescuing of the other. Not only is this behaviour emotionally unhealthy for it, as it distracts from its evolutionary growth, it prevents others from engag-ing with the lessons needed to progress on their own journey.

Home, hearth and family are critical to this Moon as a natural healing salve, along with meaningful quiet time spent with those who are dear. And yet family isn't restricted only to blood ties. To those with whom one senses a 'soul connection', a connection that feels familiar despite the ab-sence of mundane reason, these relationships are equally important.

Cancer is a hesitant sign, so this Moon isn't likely to jump out of the airplane and skydive like an Aries Moon, but it will support his or her Aries friend by happily cheer-ing them on – from the ground below! And although this Moon is extremely sensitive, with the ability to sense hurts in others, words of truth are easily expressed in supportive ways far less hurtful and damaging than is found in some of the other signs.

Symbolized in the zodiac by the Crab, which retreats into the safety of its shell at the first sign of instinctual danger, this symbol reflects Cancer's challenge. In order to grow, it must learn to push back against imagined dreads that threaten emotional and sometimes physical paralysis leading to a life of endless fearfulness.

And yet in its highest expression, the Moon's goal is to heal itself and others in ways that do no harm. By first transforming their own wounded, emotional landscape that constricts them, they then can heal others as their soul intends.

MOON IN LEO ♌

Those born with their Moon in Leo come into this life with a heart-centered generosity of spirit and, above all, a drive for creative self-expression. But the caveat for manifesting Leo's creative self-expression requires taking an emotional risk in exchange for recognition and appreciation by others. If no such risk is involved, the outward expression is simply an act that has nothing to do with an authentic self that loves to play and find joy in life.

The well-known astrologer, Dane Rudhyar (1895-1985), maintained that each of the zodiacal signs was a reaction to the excesses of the sign immediately preceding it. As we think about this, we can see that following the sensitive con-servativism of Cancer, the Leo Moon is ready to break out, roar and carry on.

Like Aries and Sagittarius, Leo Moons are of the fire element and fire likes to make things happen. Leo's evo-lutionary path is to teach the heart that it's okay to enjoy life, to play and roar without fear of repercussion – and this

Moon in its high expression likes to be big and be noticed. The possibility of leadership also waits to be tapped in this Moon. Fire Moons are sensitive to lines of power and competition around them. Keenly aware of any rivalry, real or imagined, the Leo Moon notices who's getting the attention if it isn't them. This doesn't necessarily always mean, though, that it needs to be 'performing' to be noticed. The attention it craves can come as something simple, such as a new hairstyle or outfit, noticed by another, making it 'feel' appreciated.

As with all signs, Leo's high potential can go off the rails – and when it does, this Moon retreats into an introverted armour of self-protection, not unlike Cancer retreating into its shell. The difference is that while Cancer retreats in visceral fear, Leo hides its authentic self behind a fabricated mask of superiority to reinforce its sense of place in the world. As an example, the character Hyacinth Bouquet, or Bucket, played by the brilliant Patricia Routledge in the BBC comedy series, 'Keeping Up Appearances', is a perfect example of the wheels coming off with Leo Moon.

MOON IN VIRGO ♍

On the heels of Leo's generosity and creativity comes the practical, perfectionistic Virgo Moon. A firm commitment to soul growth this lifetime rests in this Moon's evolutionary intent. Achieved through the development of a skill set in the name of service, the heart's reigning need is to make a difference in the lives of others in ways that truly matter. And whatever work is undertaken, it *must* matter. It must make a difference.

In its high expression, this Moon recognizes that in order to develop such skills and even the coveted growth it seeks, these things can't be achieved alone. This requires the search for and acceptance of, teachers and/or mentors, people travelling the same path, but are a few steps ahead, offering the essential lesson for growth: humility.

Driven by its vision of self-perfection and its place in the world, this Moon is never satisfied (which often extends to others or a situation) in its pursuit of the ideal. This comes with the challenge to face down judgmental, internal dialogue, the mental crazymakers who chatter and rail on, saying, 'this is where I should be, but this is where I am'.

Learning the art of discernment and clear self-assessment within a framework of reality is paramount for Virgo. In order to grow, this Moon must work to avoid falling into the damaging pothole of hypercriticism of the self and others when it meets life's reality head on. Steady routines, one foot in front of the other, can bring comfort to this Moon when it gets trapped on the mouse wheel of self-doubt.

MOON IN LIBRA ♎

Taking a breath after Virgo's endless pursuit of perfection, the Libra Moon at its best manifests the energy of harmony and balance for which it's known. At its heart, Libra is learning to trust and rest in tranquillity, especially when it comes to relationships and esthetic experiences.

For a Libra Moon, all forms of relationships are critical. These include not only traditional partnering such as marriage and 'significant others', but connections in business and long-term friendships as well. The give and take of emotion with another is significant for this Moon, which makes building the metaphorical bridge imperative. Libra loves the sensation of touch, so the ability to 'feel' those things deemed beautiful through its eyes is also important.

As the diplomat of the zodiac who brokers and values harmony, justice and balance, the skill of seeing both sides to a situation or disagreement, the dynamic of negotiation is innate to this Moon when it's in balance. While Libra wants everyone happy in the rowboat, this desire can swamp it.

Because of the wish for harmony, the choice of non-action has consequences. It doesn't take much for a Libra Moon to go down the rabbit hole of indecisiveness and dithering, which can easily lead to meaningless, insincere twaddle in the effort to keep everything in harmony. Telling people what they want to hear rather than what they need to hear is but one form of avoiding commitment. This rabbit hole is dangerous territory, for such non-action harbours the potential of the soul getting lost in an unrealized life.

MOON IN SCORPIO ♏

'The woods are lovely, dark and deep.
But I have promises to keep.
And miles to go before I sleep.
And miles to go before I sleep.'

These last lines from 'Stopping by the Woods on a Snowy Evening,' by the American poet Robert Frost, could easily apply to an unvarnished reflection of the Scorpio Moon.

Scorpio's evolutionary intent is always about 'miles to go' in its excavation down to the depths of its feelings in search of the authentic self. Bringing the unconscious, hidden wounds of the Scorpio heart into consciousness requires exploration of Scorpio's innermost landscape where the dragons lurk. This isn't work for the 'faint of heart'. Nor is it work typically undertaken without the help of someone skilled in assisting such an excavation who acts as a guide or witness.

As a sign that thrives on intensity, particularly in relationships, authenticity is critical for Scorpio. Only then can an emotional bond with another be established that's genuine.

When this happens, there's the reward of an emotional closeness generated by an innate, highly intuitive insight. Whether or not they're consciously aware of it, this sensitivity in those born with a Scorpio Moon is often regarded as psychic. With such sensitivity, setting emotional boundaries and privacy is important for the health of this Moon, but like all signs, Scorpio has its psychological shadow.

Scorpio can fixate on things and questions that simply have no answers. The result is obsession, throwing this Moon into depression and a darkness which feels so familiar – the underworld, the unconscious. This is particularly the case when emotionally hurt. Striking back like the Scorpion, especially in relationships, the Scorpio Moon can easily hold grudges. In such cases, self-care involves stepping back to cool off with the option of revisiting the situation for possible reconciliation or simply walking away.

MOON IN SAGITTARIUS ♐

Represented by the mythological image of a Centaur – half horse, half man, with its arrow poised to the heavens, Sagittarius is always on the quest. For those born with a Sagittarius Moon there's a deep sense of faith, sometimes unconscious, that trusts they're protected by the unseen world and laws of the Universe. While Sagittarius' quest is to discover the meaning of life, theirs in particular, this is only one layer.

For this Moon, it isn't just necessary to discover the answers it seeks unequivocally, but to drink in experiences encountered on the journey of the search, which sometimes can lead to colossal mis-steps. Nevertheless, these mis-steps aren't wasted because they add to Sagittarius' storehouse of hard-won insights. Regardless of the pros and cons, this Moon must be fed by adventure. No matter how modest or exotic, the adventure needs to be expansive and unique to them. It must be 'felt in the bones' as if stepping into a dimension that, on one hand, is out of their comfort zone but on the other, just too enticing to turn down. Whatever opportunity presents itself, there must be a richness to it with the full understanding that to take a pass through an error in judgment or exaggerated practicalities, this is saying 'no' to life.

When the Sagittarius Moon falls down the rabbit hole of its low expression, the trap of pontificating and opinionated intransigence awaits. Sadly, the goal of acquiring purposeful wisdom on its evolutionary journey is then derailed.

MOON IN CAPRICORN ♑

Amid their emotional tendency toward caution, developing personal honour, integrity, and self-discipline are the touchstones for Capricorn Moons. In order for this Moon to realize the wisdom and maturity critical to its evolutionary process, a challenging accomplishment is needed. Something striking, meaningful to this Moon, must be undertaken, and this often involves an internal process that can be equally demanding.

Still, not everyone is meant to win a Nobel Prize or to write the next bestseller. A Capricorn's enterprise can be something modest, such as volunteering at the local food bank, establishing a pet-sitting business or building that tool shed in the back garden. No matter what form such commitment takes in the process required for emotional eldership, the Capricorn heart develops and learns the lessons of self-discipline, integrity and ethical behaviour.

A cautious sign by nature, more so than any other sign in the zodiac, Capricorn is always on the alert for outside threats, real or imagined. But when the emotional energy of this Moon spools out of control into its lower expression, it sees danger everywhere. Survival is at risk. When such intense caution takes over, a 'Cap Moon' can easily get stuck in paralyzing fear.

Working quietly in measured solitude: this is restorative medicine for Capricorn. Obstacles often appear for all of us in pursuit of a goal, but setbacks can tempt this Moon to throw in the towel early, resulting in self-imposed control issues, grief, depression, unhealthy austerity, and extreme solitude. In the end, it has two choices: in pursuit of its goal, work hard to the point of exhaustion, but with satisfaction that the mountain has been climbed or do nothing and be depressed ... always a choice.

MOON IN AQUARIUS ≈

This is a rebel at heart, one that must have freedom. For those born with an Aquarian Moon, it's not a straightforward path and often comes with the feeling they're the salmon swimming upstream against the prevailing currents of society.

In order to embrace its evolutionary goal, the Aquarius Moon must honour its innate need for individuation, the honouring of its authentic self in the face of everyone having a blueprint for who it should be and how to behave. Through the eyes of others' judgment, if this Moon isn't toeing the line there's an internal sense that something's wrong with them, which can make 'staying the evolutionary course' difficult. At the slightest hint of its uniqueness being compromised, as this square peg tries to fit into a round hole, the Aquarius Moon can feel as if it's being shoved into a straitjacket.

By honouring what feels right in their heart, the risk for subjects of this Moon is that people will leave – and some will, triggering the possibility of regret or grief for a time. But going along with the flow, agreeing to something which contradicts the authentic self, dishonours the heart. Conversely, resisting just for the sake of resisting, rejecting compromise in order to hold on to a vision – then a life of loneliness and disassociation may lie on the path ahead. The challenge then is to find the balance of one foot in each canoe.

Aquarian Moons thrive on 'making it up as they go along'; they're eccentrics more often than not, their make-up perhaps flavoured with a good dose of wackiness. But the rest of us should not be fooled, for these souls who love exchanging ideas and methods that shatter entrenched margins frequently emerge as our visionary geniuses. Without them, we'd still be wearing animal skins.

MOON IN PISCES ♓

We now come to the last sign in the zodiac, dreamy Pisces – whose heart belongs not to the ego but to the soul and spiritual realm. Pisces Moons aren't complicated. In its high expression, this Moon can engage with the outer world and yet maintain its primal connection with Spirit more than any other sign.

Creative endeavours such as painting, dance, writing, playing or listening to music, to name just a few examples, support this Moon's connection to its core essence. Visionary seeds are often planted when such pursuits are genuinely engaged in. It's almost as if the individual shifts into a trans-state, crossing the invisible boundary between dimensions. Leonardo da Vinci, Michelangelo and Coco Chanel, visionaries all, were born with their Moon in Pisces.

As we learned earlier, our Moon, no matter what sign it's in, is naturally sensitive. But with Pisces (along with the other two water signs, Cancer and Scorpio), this sensitivity is heightened. Born with unconditional compassion, they may find it near impossible to stem the tide of ambient emotions around them. As if they're a small boat being tossed about on turbulent waters, addictions to dampen the pain of feeling too much lurk as an undercurrent – in dragon territory. Imaginative creativity, states of calm, a daily quiet time and Dr Bach's remedies are among self-care strategies. With Pisces, the ever-present alternative is going down the rabbit hole of a lifetime filled with unproductive behaviours and truncated evolution.

ELEVEN

—

More than a Memory

The past is never where you think you left it.
Katherine Anne Porter

BACK IN Chapter Nine, we were introduced to the early history and philosophy behind Evolutionary Astrology, with its psychological lens anchored in the concept that our goal is to evolve at the soul level. Through this lens, we recognize that every planet, sign and placement is a thread in the divine web of the soul, woven against the backdrop of the universe. Through these threads we see patterns that make up the emotional condition of the soul as it incarnated into this physical life.

Western astrology uses a great many symbols in a chart, and among these are symbols for the Moon's 'Nodes'. From the evolutionary perspective, their placement and relationship to our natal planets are critical in identifying unresolved emotional karma carried forward into this incarnation.

Represented by symbols for the Moon's north/south nodal axis, this emotional karma has now 'ripened'. And it's through these symbols, as we learned earlier, that our soul is telling us we're ready to deal with whatever behaviour, attitude or responses were present in past circumstances that hung us up. As the universe is perfect in its orchestration, those circumstances with their underlying emotions have now reappeared, although updated, giving us the opportunity to 'switch the channel'. The choice is ours.

So where does the nodal axis lie in our chart? To answer this, we can look at another sample chart.

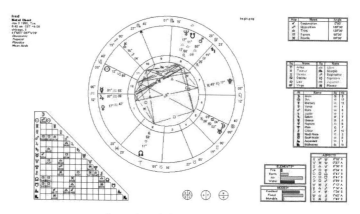

Screenshot of Astrodienst sample chart with the North Node

In the chart sample itself, near the bottom of the planet list, in the third table to the right of the chart wheel, you'll see the notation, 'North Node' with a symbol that looks like an upright 'horseshoe', ☊, in the sign of Aries. In this sample chart we find it placed in the second house at the bottom. Conversely, your chart always contains a 'South Node' represented by what looks like an upside down horseshoe exactly opposite in position and sign from the north. In our example, the South Node appears in the sign of Libra, in the eighth house, upper right corner of the chart.

Although these are the symbols for the Moon's nodes, what are they, really, and why are they important? As Steven Forrest points out, 'Physically the nodes … are moving points that have to do with the relationship of the Moon's orbit to the celestial sphere…. [But] for our purposes we do not need to understand them in scientific terms. It is their symbolic meaning we must grasp.'*

*Steven Forrest, THE INNER SKY, 1985 p. 211

Charts cast using the Astrodienst website referred to in Chapter Nine do not reflect the Moon's South Node symbol, which is critical and always opposite the North Node symbol. While a different resource has been used for this discussion, it's a non-public resource. For this reason I've included a table of the nodal pairings here for reference. To find your South Node, simply look to the column across from the North Node.

NODAL PAIRINGS

NORTH NODE	*SOUTH NODE*
ARIES	LIBRA
TAURUS	SCORPIO
GEMINI	SAGITTARIUS
CANCER	CAPRICORN
LEO	AQUARIUS
VIRGO	PISCES
LIBRA	ARIES
SCORPIO	TAURUS
SAGITTARIUS	GEMINI
CAPRICORN	CANCER
AQUARIUS	LEO
PISCES	VIRGO

The nodal symbolism in a chart and what it represents comes with ancient roots in Vedic Astrology, the system used in India. In Vedic work, the nodes are referred to as *ketu*, the Dragon's Tail (south) and *rahu*, Dragon's Head (north). Once again, the importance of our dragons appears! In modern times with the emergence of Evolutionary Astrology, nodal symbolism has come to the forefront of importance in the western system.

The South Node, ☋, in our chart represents us in a past life and the piece of the unresolved emotional karma that's travelled forward with us for reconciliation in the present. This karma may be from a most recent past life or further back. The actual stories behind our long line of prior lifetimes don't really matter. What does matter is that 'something went amiss' and that the emotions involved in a particular experience, or collection of experiences, have come up for review as a critical piece in the discovery of our evolutionary purpose. The good news is that coming into this incarnation, we now have internal resources to confront the unresolved emotions involved and to transform them if we choose to do so. *And* in our process, we also have the external support of Dr Bach's remedies to help us. However, again it's important to remember that specific remedy choices depend very much on how one experiences nuances of the negative emotions brought forward for healing. For example, lack of courage can drive the emotion of fear when facing down a threat or it can result from simply lacking self-confidence – two very different scenarios.

Let's return to our sample chart with the path to ☊ North Node's healing medicine placed opposite of ☋, the South Node. Make no mistake, while we'd like to think it as such, this journey to the north isn't a quick trip; it's a lifetime's amount of work, as is our evolution. In this it's important to remember that while the unresolved emotions remain, the circumstances of the life or lives responsible for creating the unresolved karma are in the past; it's over and done. Still, an Evolutionary Astrologer can see footprints from the past in a chart by studying the nodal axis and planetary connections to it. Through this analysis, he or she can ascertain the residual negative emotions which have come forth for review and transformation as part of the chart's story.*

Although the focus for Evolutionary Astrologers is with a negative eye cast to the past, the South Node's karmic emotions include, to a lesser degree, positive emotions. Still, it's the emotions in need of transformation that come to the head of the line. And, as these are worked with, we can take comfort in knowing that, yes, we have also carried forward positive qualities stored in our emotional karmic bank account as a much-needed resource in this incarnation.

Proper analysis of the nodal story in a chart is a complicated process involving many factors and steps in teasing out the threads of the past, evaluating what went wrong and possible resolutions in the present. It's important to recognize that the quality of analysis depends on a combination of the astrologer's training, experience and, to some extent, intuitive abilities. Nevertheless, through my own lens, which is certainly not exclusive, let's take a brief look at the nodal axis in Bach's own chart.

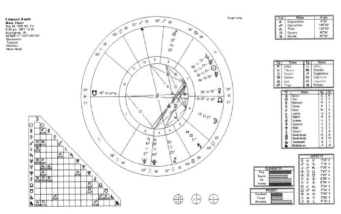

Screenshot of Bach's own chart from Astrodienst

*Note: Sometimes, depending on the astrologer's training, she or he will wrap the symbolism of the South Node around a metaphorical story for easier understanding of what occurred in creating the karmic footprint.

At a passing glance, we can see that the South Node of his Moon rests in the twelfth house, in Pisces. Among several interpretations for this sign and house are those of the mystic and spiritualism. It's important to note that interpretations of houses and signs are infinite, which is why taking into account the symbols and placements of the entire chart is so important; everything is connected, usually revealing one or more repetitive themes. However, with this look at the South Node in Bach's chart, we immediately know something went wrong for him in the lifetime up for review, having to do with his spiritual perceptions and circumstances, as reflected by the chart's symbol placements.* Although this is only the beginning, this is where we start to unravel his story, one having to do with the desire to establish a *rapport* with the Divine. The question is, what went wrong for him back then? Based on the symbol placements and therefore with a fair amount of certainty, we start with the notion that Bach lost his way and himself amidst his spiritual calling in that life.

In Evolutionary Astrology, the twelfth house also denotes loss, including dissolution of the ego. One of the possibilities is that as an ecstatic, Bach simply slipped off the plate, emotionally. Earlier, we saw a manifestation of such dissociation in the discussion concerning 'holy anorexia' in medieval nunneries. I'm not suggesting this was the situation in Bach's case (as it was also evident in the monasteries), but only as an example of how a continued state of ecstasy can result in people's 'losing themselves'. This aside,

*In IGNITING SOUL FIRE : SPIRITUAL DIMENSIONS OF THE BACH FLOWER REMEDIES, I offered an account of Bach's chart using an unverified time of birth. Since then, an alternative chart has emerged for purposes of this discussion. As with the prior chart in IGNITING, Bach's birth time is not officially verified but sourced from possible rectification. Bach was born in Moseley, UK, a suburb of Birmingham.

because of the spiritual ego-loss and ramifications with the South Node in the twelfth, an exceedingly complex picture almost always emerges as the chart's planetary relationships to this node are considered. Far beyond the scope of this discussion, were we to dive more deeply into this chart, we could weave the fabric of a metaphorical story revealing the psychological motivations driving Bach's unresolved karma into the life we know.

But what about his healing on the path forward? In a proper chart analysis of the nodal axis, we look to energetic patterns connected to the North Node as the way forward. In a very limited examination of Bach's healing journey, we can see with the sixth house North Node in Virgo, opposite the twelfth, his healing evolutionary goal this time around was to walk a path of service. The intention here was not to function as a 'servant' but to be in service to something through work that mattered, involving the development of a grounded skill set with the help of mentors and teachers. It's no surprise then, to learn that among these resources for Bach were the early nineteenth-century written teachings of Samuel Hahnemann, the father of Homeopathy. By following the path of medicine, this was the way forward for Bach to heal the ungrounded ecstasy and escapism that the chart indicates may have dominated his past. It's also no accident that, among other things, the sixth house is tied to healing and health.

Even though the primary focus of our nodal story up for examination is concerned with what 'went wrong' in the past, it's important to recall that we also carry forward elements of positivity. In Bach's case, this positivity rests in his heightened mystical and spiritual gifts, critical components behind his discovery of the thirty-eight flower remedies.

In the next chapter we focus on a closer look at the

South Node by sign, beginning once again with Aries. And, as we explore this territory, we can consider the virtues of Dr Bach's remedies as a support on the journey of reconciling unresolved emotional karma – and perhaps how it appears in our own chart.

TWELVE

—

Switching the Channel

*'If you don't follow your nature, there's a hole in the
Universe where you were supposed to be.'*
Dane Rudhyar

AS WE DIVE further into the territory of the lunar
South Node, it's useful to note that overlap will appear in the descriptive energies for each of the signs,
but with nuances. In the energy of Aries, for example, both
the high and low expressions are ever a consideration. The
differences lie in the subtleties of the circumstances and application. You can put lipstick on a pig, but at its core, it's
still a pig. The question that always arises when focusing on
a chart's nodal axis is, what is the course correction needed
to move forward in this lifetime? There's not always an easy
answer but the journey is part of our evolutionary work and
within it, the need to recognize we're now strong enough
to confront what went wrong before and to work toward
the higher expression of the emotions involved, this time
around, especially with the help of Dr Bach's remedies.

A final reminder on this process is that in practice, an
Evolutionary Astrologer would discuss the energy found
in the North Node sign and specifics regarding the client's
healing pathway. While with some of the signs I've loosely
referred to the North's energies (without naming the North's
signs) I've not gone into depth with the pairings. My reason-
ing for this is twofold. Primary is my intent to focus on the

South Node. The core premise of this book is how we can discover our evolutionary purpose through an awareness of imbalanced emotions, whether looking at them through Dr Bach's lens, the lens of Evolutionary Astrology or imbalances in the energy of our chakras. Within the framework of Evolutionary Astrology, we consider that from a significant prior incarnation, we carry forward emotions holding us up on our evolutionary journey. This is the reason they're outlined in the negative descriptions.

I also want to re-emphasize that, as I pointed out in the brief discussion of Dr Bach's chart, the nodal axis puzzle is complex. For example, a South Node in Virgo can indicate something more than just the individual being hard on themselves (and others) by not doing or being 'enough'. Certainly this is 'part of the story' – it's just not all of it. While the range of possibilities, including the extreme ones, isn't to point fingers of guilt, its purpose is to highlight the fact that these negative emotions, regardless of the depth of manifestation, are hindrances (to use Dr Bach's term) to our process. Examples are given, again not for readers to identify with but to point up the work that can be done.

And there is good news. Through our chart's symbols, we're also put on notice that we've evolved far enough and have the tools within us to meet these hindrances head on, to transform them into their 'highest expression' – their state of virtue – propelling us further along on our very important evolutionary journey. A little bit of shorthand is the result only of the practical matter of space. Nevertheless, it's hoped that in these descriptions, clues as to which of Dr Bach's remedies might be useful in switching your own channel should you have access to your chart and nodal axis, will emerge. For those unfamiliar with the positive and negative states for each of Dr Bach's thirty-eight remedies, resources are listed under the 'Further Reading' section. Additionally, while there are hundreds of possible combinations of Dr Bach's thirty-eight, I have offered a few remedy suggestions at the end of each nodal entry. Additionally, it's important to keep in mind that the primary focus is the characteristic of the particular emotions described rather than the metaphorical story.

SOUTH NODE ARIES ♈

If we see an Aries South Node in our chart, we know coming up for consideration is a prior life or possibly more than one lifetime, in which we were under a great deal of tension and pressure. In the earlier discussion concerning an Aries natal Moon, we remembered that Mars was the god of war in Roman mythology. In western astrology every zodiacal sign has a planetary ruler, and for Aries, it's Mars. If we consider the intense energy of Mars ruling the South Node, we can be fairly certain the nature of our stress was emotional, and often physical as well, depending on the circumstances.

We also know that when it comes to Aries, we can be fairly confident in assuming we were in a situation involving intense conflict – most likely it wasn't just one incident but ongoing circumstances, dominated by some form of violence we were forced to deal with.

While it's impossible to know for certain what these circumstances were, we can speculate on possibilities depending on where the South Node falls in the chart and connections to the other planets. Were we a soldier on the battlefield? Were we a mother without privilege, struggling to protect our family as war raged throughout the city? Or were we a victim in an emotionally abusive situation? The possibilities are vast, and because they are – as with all South Node placements – what we want to concentrate on is the emotional damage we were unable to overcome in the past.

This brings us to our healing path of transforming the disturbing ravages of Aries. From this past life or lives, we came into this world frightened and possibly angry down to our bones. There's a need, then, to heal the fear, rage, and kneejerk reactions to perceived dangers and or aggression. Remember, that past life is now over. We need peace and love in order to move forward. We need to work on connecting to those with whom we can share a bond, a bond we can sink into without fear or anger, but with trust. This goal is part of our soul's agenda.

Suggested remedies: Holly, Mimulus, Rock Rose, Willow

SOUTH NODE TAURUS ♉

Not every past-life experience is filled with high drama, where we were burned at the stake for bucking the system! There are lives in which we opted for safe inaction and simplicity because it was easier, uncomplicated, and far more attractive than facing the complexities of life on offer.

Such is the case with the South Node in Taurus. As we noted earlier, by its nature Taurean emotional energy desires stability, security and is cautious. No drama. But from an evolutionary perspective, becoming entrenched in conservatism, opting for doing things the way they've always been done, doesn't do much in terms of progress. This particularly might be the case if our family traditions and expectations have been put on a pedestal, the world views that come with these not to be questioned. As we know, times change for the better, more often than not. Applications and expectations that worked in the past might be so far out of date that, if we're honest with ourselves, they don't even appear in our rear-view mirror as practical for our soul's growth.

With this South Node, our sole concern in the past focused on keeping life on an even keel, avoiding unpleasantness at all costs, even if facing these things down would have been to our advantage. By going along to get along, settling for less than, avoiding the possibility of the unexpected, the cost of our passivity led to a kind of laziness. Tradition and conservatism aren't necessarily a bad thing unless this overshadows every aspect of our being, keeping us stuck, keeping ourselves and life predictable. The potential outcomes of acquiescence are vast.

This time around, our soul is challenging us specifically to own and come to terms with our core emotions---no more glossing over, no more sidestepping. Our evolutionary agenda is to dive deep. What does our heart really want? To answer this question, we're being challenged to commit to an excavation of our emotions, to acknowledge what psychology calls our shadow by digging into the muck of our humanness – those things which Dr Bach said 'vex us': our jealousies, greed, misguided passions. When we make peace with them, when we let go of them by transforming them through this excavation as part of who we are, then we're able to engage with life as we're meant to for our highest and greatest potential.

Suggested remedies: Rock Water, Vine, Walnut

SOUTH NODE GEMINI ♊

With the South Node Gemini, we know we're looking at a life in which our mental quickness was paramount. Ruled by quicksilver Mercury, 'messenger of the gods' who represents the mind, language and communication, Gemini oversees our perception of the world. With a look to the past, our thought processes most likely served us well in rapidly changing circumstances requiring agile adaptability

– until we got into trouble.

And of course, because we're dealing with the South Node, how we went down the rabbit hole varies widely. One of the possibilities is that perhaps we were known for our superior intellect. However, because of our telescoped focus, from our ivory tower in the head, we missed opportunities … the phrase 'can't see the wood for the trees' has a familiar ring!

On the night of April 14th 1912, Edward Smith, Captain of the doomed ocean liner, *Titanic*, willingly ignored warnings of icebergs in the area from seven other ships. He wilfully forged ahead at full speed, refusing all advice to change course. In this case, the familiar expression used by sailors, 'hold the course', led to one of history's greatest nautical disasters. Because of his disregard of the bigger picture, which required mental lightning reflexes in consideration of the dangerous circumstances, 1,200 souls were lost in the Atlantic's icy waters.

Or maybe, unlike Captain Smith, we weren't in such a lofty position. Instead, we were in circumstances where every day we faced life or death. Perhaps because of our nefarious behaviours and cleverness we caught the eye of Elizabeth I's spymaster, Sir Francis Walsingham. Although we initially escaped the noose under Walsingham's protection, our life was under the constant stress of a double-edged sword in avoiding mis-steps. Get Walsingham's assignment wrong and we died amid carrying it out – or in opting for mental, scattered reflexes instead of a predominant strategy, we failed, losing Walsingham's protection.

Nevertheless, a Gemini South Node doesn't necessarily suggest a dire ending. The bigger issue is that in the past our circumstances required constant improvization in the mist of turmoil. In this incarnation the key is to recognize that in order to heal the penchant for mental dominance, we're called to stretch our horizons, consider exploring unfamiliar territories temporally or perhaps philosophically. In the spirit of our evolutionary progress, it's time to widen our scope beyond the end of our nose. Explore the possibilities, integrate our mental swiftness from the past with innate faith and intuition in the present.

Suggested remedies: Cerato, Larch

SOUTH NODE CANCER ♋

As indicated in Chapter Ten, Cancer is the Great Mother of the zodiac. Feeling so deeply, with its heightened sensitivity, those with a Cancer South Node come from a past in which they had little or no emotional filter. Carried forward is an abundant tendency to intervene and rescue in ways that are well-meant, but in reality are unhelpful to the 'other'. Ranging from mild to extreme, there are many examples of how this behaviour manifests.

Recalling that Cancer is tied to the concept of family – blood and otherwise – one excessive instance would be the 'helicoptering parent', a kind of modern 'stage mother' who overmanages her child in the hopes of a successful rise to prominence. A poignant illustration is the well-publicized contemporary career of child star, Brooke Shields. Her distressing early years were managed with an iron fist by an emotionally troubled mother, something Shield talks about in her autobiography, *There was a Little Girl*.

However, misguided, other-directed overcare isn't the only unresolved issue possible for a South Node Cancer. We might have been in circumstances that triggered feelings our needs weren't being met or paid attention to. What about a woman forced into a marriage of convenience for the sake of her family's fortunes? Or conversely, what about a man forced into a contractual marriage and yet in love with another woman – or man?

Such events can prompt a familiar retreat into the Cancerian shell. When this happens, we can become so focused on our inner landscape of insufferable self-pity, that it buries the innate gift of caring for others in the spirit of 'doing no harm'. Whining, whingeing or launching into emotional drama in order to get attention may show their ugly head.

While it sounds somewhat harsh, the expression 'pull up your socks' reflects the evolutionary course-correction in the present incarnation for a Cancer South Node. In order to leave the emotional past behind, it's time to grow up, step into maturity and set boundaries. The instinct to 'care' remains, but it needs tempering. Otherwise, those who are the object of the 'overcare' will never be accountable for their own behaviour and consequences. And they'll continue to suck the life out of their rescuers.

Suggested remedies: Chicory, Heather, Willow

SOUTH NODE LEO ♌

If the South Node in our chart has landed in Leo, a possibility is that we're looking at a prior life in which we were royalty – or, at the very least, privileged. At first glance, this seems a pretty good deal. Who wouldn't like to be at the head of the pecking order?

However, with this South Node we can be fairly certain that we found ourselves in a golden cage of some ilk – all that's gold doesn't always glitter. As an example, we can look to the circumstances under which Britain's King George VI came to the throne in 1936. Thrown into this position because of his brother's abdication in order to marry Wallace Simpson, King George found himself in circumstances he did not expect and which some believe led to his premature death.

If we're looking at royalty (which is one possibility, but

at the least, privilege or leadership in some fashion) through a Leo South Node, we know that expectations, through the eyes of society, dictated our behaviour. Regardless of the specifics, we were somehow the object of admiration which led to our attitude. No matter the degree of veneration, we grew to like this feeling directed toward us, but it came with 'hindrances', to use Dr Bach's terminology. Perhaps it was arrogance, a selfishness or maybe the love of creating drama around us that fed our desire, our need for approval. The list is long, but nevertheless we developed a susceptibility to an insatiable grasping that sabotaged our authentic self.

In this present incarnation, the path to healing a Leo South Node is through finding one's individuation, tempering that need for adulation. This journey requires gaining release from the constraints of other's expectations. In order to succeed, it requires taking risks that expose our authenticity – taking risks of exposure that bear an uncertain outcome. Such action doesn't fall into that easy realm where lawyers only ask questions to which they know the answers. This is the realm of taking a leap of faith in ourselves.

Suggested remedies: Gentian, Larch

SOUTH NODE VIRGO ♍

If we see the South Node in Virgo in our chart, most likely we were someone under the threat of emotional breakdown because of our chronic attempts to be perfect and to manifest perfection in everything we attempted. In reality, what *is* perfection and by whose measures can we gauge it?

In the earlier discussion concerning the evolutionary intent of a Virgo Moon, we noted that as a sign, Virgo is never satisfied. For a Virgo South Node, this emotional state in a past life or lives up for examination was constant. Deep within us, we've carried this burden into the present incarnation.

Never being satisfied with the self is an open invitation to chronic self-judgment and low self-esteem. In short, we're never enough, never going to be enough, unless we undertake a course correction to switch the channel. The emotional shroud of self-determined failure and inadequacy is heavy.

This raises the question as to what triggered a self-inflicted punishing attitude? Looking into the past, one possibility is a misguided sense of inescapable duty to others stemming from insecurity and loss of a balanced perspective. Another possibility is that we were a disciple in the orbit of a false guru who was abusive emotionally, sexually or both. And then there's always the prospect of hierarchal expectation.

Regardless of the exact circumstances, we've carried forward some shame and guilt … the dark twins who keep on giving, bleeding the joy of this life out of us. The counterbalance is to 'let go and let God' (Spirit, the Divine, or whatever term you're comfortable with) in the understanding that the higher realm doesn't care about our obsessive grasps and deceptive goal of perfection. With the help of Dr Bach's remedies, we can come to a place of understanding that by surrendering to unconditional love of the Divine, we are worthy of breathing fresh air, saying YES to life.

Suggested remedies: Beech, Crab Apple, Pine,

SOUTH NODE LIBRA ♎

Many years ago, a psychotherapist friend of mine made this remark over dinner: 'Relationships are tricky and difficult, no matter who's involved'. She was right. As humans, we're a complex of emotions driven by our desires, wrapped up in a physical body. And, unless we're living solo on a desert island or at the far edge of the polar outback, engaging with others is part of our package in this incarnation, where we span a vast landscape of relationships.

As noted earlier, Libra is often referred to as the diplomat of the zodiac, opting for harmony and balance, very different from Aries who forges ahead, the torpedoes be damned. If the South Node shows up in Libra with its predilection for harmony and balance in relationships, we need to recognize there were times and situations when this was too much of a good thing. As with all the signs, there are limitless possibilities in how this dynamic played out. But for certain, we were in circumstances in which our wellbeing, such as it might have been, required pleasing another or others in order to keep the peace (and sometimes our head) at all costs.

Were we a courtesan in the court of Louis XIV or part of a Raj prince's harem, where our elevated status could tumble in a heartbeat? It's possible. However, there's also the possibility that circumstances were not so elevated and pampered. Perhaps we ended up in America in the 1600s from across the Atlantic to live the life of an indentured servant or an African slave. Whatever the case, our quality of life and often our very survival depended on us being subservient in ways that kept whomsoever was holding the strings of our life happy.

The course correction from that life or lives requires us to adopt determination in claiming our independence, stopping the placating, embracing the pure will and courage to set boundaries and ability to say 'No'.

Suggested remedies: Centaury, Chestnut Bud, Walnut

SOUTH NODE SCORPIO ♏

As human beings, there are truly awful things that happen to us, things that trigger panic attacks complete with hyperventilation and cold sweats in the middle of the night. With this South Node, the relevant past has seen us as either victim or perpetrator, embroiled in a kind of diabolical horror. But what actually happened? As noted earlier, it's impossible to pinpoint exactly, but in order to consider possibilities, we require a lot more information. Although I'll give some colourful examples, sometimes our trauma was something unapparent to others.

What we can determine, however, is that our circumstances were atrocious. On the rack as a guest of the Inquisition? Starved to death in a Nazi prison camp or on the Bataan Death March? Any of these scenarios are quite possible, as is the chance of our being on the other side of the coin. Whatever happened, we know emotional intensity was part of the scenario and the circumstances a complex of dark waters that left wounds of trauma on our soul.

Nevertheless, through it all, we've brought forward hardwon wisdom. But in order to heal from those cellular memories, we need to ground ourselves into the body, even though our gut instinct prefers we do anything but that. Still, it's the only way. We need to calm down. We need peace in mind, body and soul. We need circumstances in which we feel enveloped by well-meant, tangible intentions from others and at the very least, surround ourselves in an environment of things natural and of an earthly nature. This is the panacea that can bring us up into the light from the 'dark night of the soul' in that Scorpio lifetime.

Suggested remedies: Aspen, Mimulus, Star of Bethlehem, Sweet Chestnut

SOUTH NODE SAGITTARIUS ♐

Coming up from the depths of Scorpio, Sagittarius launches into its endless quest to grasp the meaning of life, usually with an exuberance for adventure and experience. We met

Sagittarius earlier in the discussion surrounding the evolutionary meanings behind the signs of the natal Moon and yet, with this South Node, there isn't an awful lot that's different except for falling down the rabbit hole in a prior life.

With this South Node, we were wired in that past life to make spectacular miscalculations in our worldview and we got stuck, likely in areas that had to do with established religion or a prevailing belief system. Perhaps we were card-carrying members of the Flat Earth Society! Perhaps we were among the Jesuits who charged Galileo with heresy, condemning his astronomical theories.

As we land in this incarnation we've brought along our blanket of rigidity surrounding those prior beliefs with the surety they're written in stone and our absolute truth. But in reality, this inflexibility isn't doing us any favours. It slams the door shut on the prospect of open-minded curiosity and the engagement of listening, elements necessary for shifts in perception for our evolutionary course-correction. With a Sagittarius South Node, the gauntlet has been thrown down, pressing us to change our track, to widen our curiosity outside of our rigid beliefs – with an open mind, through conversation and the willingness to listen and learn in order to chart a new course on our quest. In this way we can become both student and teacher.

Suggested remedies: Rock Water, Vine, Vervain

SOUTH NODE CAPRICORN ♑

Survival in the face of a stark and often painful circumstances is the hallmark of this South Node. In that prior life, we faced challenging options – choices that would have let us 'take a pass in doing the right thing'. And yet, at the end of the day, we did do the right We didn't whine, we stepped up to the plate and 'just got on with it' in ways that allowed us to live with our consciences.

Recalling that the nature of Capricorn tends to be solitary – from the discussion concerning the evolutionary intent of a Capricorn Moon (see pp 103-4) – most likely we were forced to act alone. With this South Node signature, it's safe to say life was difficult and probably considered dangerous. As such, we found ourselves confronted with pressing responsibilities that demanded maturity and a stoicism in the face of our reality. Despite the details of that lifetime or those lifetimes, we were reliable and could be counted upon.

Perhaps we were solely responsible for our family amid the most devastating circumstances, or maybe we held a prominent position in a community that depended upon our leadership and wise decisions in times of war. Uneasy is the head that wears the crown. Such obligation can be depressing – exhausting mind, body and soul.

In this lifetime we have come in to exhale, to find respite and healing – to let go of our stoicism and control issues. We now have permission to embrace our humanness with its fragilities as well as our brilliance. We only have to let go and admit self-nurturing, nurturing from others and gentleness into this life.

Suggested remedies: Star of Bethlehem, Rock Water

SOUTH NODE AQUARIUS ≈

Living in the head, where it's safe, rather than risking our heart's creative passion – this is the refuge for an Aquarian South Node. Whatever circumstances we found ourselves in with this node in the past, we had ideas and beliefs that bucked against the prevailing collective's agenda at the time. Were we a heretic? Certainly this is a strong consideration in the offering. But heresy or at least dissenting against the prevailing societal codes comes in many guises. Imagine what we endured if we were a secret female student of Leonardo's – at a time when it was forbidden for women to practice the arts?

There's also the possibility we were part of a movement. Perhaps we belonged to a group of like-minded souls hell-bent on a particular mission to change the world – one that was unpopular with the prevailing societal agenda. In the not-too-distant past we might have been a Suffragette lobbying for women to be given the right to vote, only to find that for all of our work, for our beliefs and efforts, we were beaten and jailed. The theory on time spent between incarnations continues to be debated, so it's possible. Regardless of our circumstances, because of our declarations we were dismissed, laughed at and most likely expelled from society, even if we didn't lose our head.

Ostracized, visionaries and radicals often end up living a lonely life. In our way-back past, our passionate, radical vision fuelled a self-inflicted attitude of such extreme rebelliousness that we lost sight of ourselves, ending up disconnected from those around us. Most importantly, we disconnected from our creative heart, a heart in need of healing this time around.

Innovation always requires creativity in some form, whether you're a writer, an actor, scientist or engineer. In order for our dreams to receive the breath of life, the head must make room for the heart and this requires taking the risk of failure before success.

When J. K. Rowling wrote HARRY POTTER AND THE PHILOSOPHER'S STONE in coffee shops, because she couldn't afford to heat her flat and was nearly destitute with a young daughter, mainstream publishers wouldn't give her the time of day. Nevertheless, she persevered, trusting her heart to take the required risk – and we know how that trust worked out.

Suggested remedies: Cerato, Gentian, Walnut

SOUTH NODE PISCES ♓

In the previous chapter we had a peek at Dr Bach's chart with his karmic South Node sitting in the house of the mystic. We now have come full course around the zodiac to dreamy Pisces, the sign of compassion, spirituality and ego-lessness. As we saw with Bach's chart, losing a sense of self, a sense of being untethered to the reality of life, was a distinctive possibility for him – which is true for those of us with this Piscean South Node placement.

Whatever the circumstances, we can be fairly certain a misguided sense of what it meant to be 'spiritual' was involved at the foundation of our emotional karma up for review. As suggested earlier, perhaps we were one of those anorexic nuns (or monks!) back in the twelfth century. In the midst of our ill-advised concept of 'service', we were convinced that the more we marginalized our physical body, the closer to the Divine we'd be, maybe recognized as a 'Special Servant of God's'.

The irony around our erroneous concept of divine service can be found in the words of an ancient Egyptian prayer: 'God grant that today I do work that matters'.* In other words, in order to perform work in the sense of spiritual service that matters on the earthly plane, we must be grounded and present in the body, the next stop on our journey of discovery.

Suggested remedies: Clematis, Wild Rose

*This is a phrase often used by Steven Forrest in his writings and in his apprenticeship teaching; so simple, yet powerful.

THIRTEEN

---

*The Seven Sacred Gates of Soul awareness: the Chakras**

SOME SAY that the eyes are the windows to the soul. But in various spiritual teachings and ancient mystery schools, it's the chakras that are considered gateways, or portals, to our soul's wisdom.

Among the many aspects of Bach's thoughts throughout his writings are those that bring his spiritual nature to light. Through these, he informs us that in addition to his relationship with the remedies he had a deep connection to those things he considered divinely inspired, including philosophies of the East. On more than one occasion, regarding a variety of subjects, Bach refers to the teachings of 'the Lord Buddha', 'Our Mother India', and to 'Masters'. He places these references within the context of their importance to healing, in that how we live – and the spiritual process used to do so – helps us to discover our soul-agenda:

> *We have the glorious example, the great standard of perfection and the teachings of The Christ to guide us.... His mission on earth was to teach us how to obtain harmony and communication with our Higher Self.... Thus also taught the Lord Buddha and other great Masters, who have come down from time to time upon earth to point out to men the way to attain perfection....†*

*Portions of this chapter were originally published in The International Journal of the Sacred Space Foundation, Fall 2003

†Barnard, COLLECTED WRITINGS, p. 156

Although absolute evidence does not seem to be available, it's reasonable to presume that among the various facets of these philosophies Bach developed a working knowledge of the 'chakras'.

The identification of the chakras is anchored in the ancient yogic tradition of Hinduism and, later, Buddhism. We may find through our sacred shopping a plethora of authoritative works about the chakras: what they are, what they do, and how they affect us. As always in discussions of spiritual beliefs, there are subtle variances in philosophy. No less is true when one considers the chakras and their relationship to 'auras'. In esoteric traditions, it's generally accepted that there's an 'envelope' of vital energy radiating from everything in nature, including the human body, known as an aura. To clairvoyants, auras manifest as energetic layers of colours. These layers surrounding the body continuously expand and contract in the intensity of their colours and in their boundaries. Interestingly, the concept of auras and energy actually dates back to the ancient world, appearing 'in the writings and art of Egypt, India, Greece, and Rome where saints appear wreathed with haloes. In the sixteenth century, Paracelsus was one of the first western scholars to expound upon the astral body, which he described as a fiery globe'.*

Recalling from Chapter Two, fundamental to the concept of chakras is that they function as seven major centres in addition to hundreds of minor ones, of continuous, vibrational energy. Operating within the 'auras' of our etheric, astral and mental bodies, they have a relationship to our physical body through the pathways of our central nervous system, which lies along our spinal column.

*HARPER'S ENCYCLOPAEDIA OF MYSTICAL AND PARANORMAL EXPERIENCE, p. 40

When we move into states of distress, consciously or unconsciously, the negative energy of our emotions initiates patterns of contraction within the chakras and our auras. Like the pebble tossed into a pond of still water, this action perpetuates disruptive permutations that reverberate throughout these layers. Spiritual writings and philosophy of the East teach us that ultimately blockages to positive energetic flow eventually manifest in illness and disease. Conversely, when we experience positive emotional states, the chakras intensify and expand into harmonic balance.

As spirit in body, our soul is constantly pushing us toward such a harmony within and amongst these centres, with the goal of bringing them into full expansion and expression for our highest good. This process of soul growth is one that leads us through the delicate intricacies of emotional balance between needing connection and courage, choice and resilience, self-love and unconditional love, emotional voice and authority, and insight and faith. Negative emotional imprints within the chakras with their vibrations and energy not only encourage a contraction from soul connection but, conversely, positive emotional imprints facilitate expansion toward the soul, within a process fluid as mercury. In working with these images, we find that the emotional imprints of the chakras are excellent maps for discovering unexplored territory. In this way, the nature of our emotions both positive and negative is cellular fuel.

When our emotions shut down, or we're emotionally 'stuck', the vibration within the chakras enters a state of contraction, resulting in operational shaky ground or no foundation at all. In order to bring our chakras into states of expansion, our emotional excavation needs to begin by exploring where we become emotionally stuck and why. Further, and most importantly, what tools do we have at our disposal to assist us in our endeavours to move out of our toxic spaces? It is here that we can look at the energetic imprints of the seven chakras and their relationship to the Bach remedies.

When we recall that the core of Bach's philosophy on the nature of healing focused on the relationship between polar opposites, the connection between the positive energy of the remedies and negative or contracted states of the chakras becomes clear – as he states:

> *If a patient has a mental [emotional] error, a conflict between physical and spiritual self will result, and disease will be the product. The error may be repelled, the poison driven from the body, but a vacuum is left, an adverse force has gone, but a space exists where it has been situated.*
>
> *The perfect method is not so much to repel the adverse influence, as to draw in its opposing virtue; and by means of this virtue, flood out the fault. This is the law of opposites, of positive and negative.* *

Taking this perspective a step further, as has been suggested in the chapters regarding the South Node placement in our astrological birth chart, the positive energy or vibrations of the remedies are capable of catalysing subtle but broad transformations within the many and often complex layers of our emotions. Thus, appropriate combinations of the remedies shift as our internal perspectives shift, facilitating an ongoing expansion of our chakras and changes in our external behaviours.

As we've already seen, Bach had a fascination with numbers and, it appears, with certain numbers in particular. Keeping in mind that there are seven major chakras, this number repeatedly appears in Bach's work. Between 1928 and 1930, he initially worked out identifying characteristics

*Barnard, COLLECTED WRITINGS, p.159

of seven behavioural groups he felt were keys to an individual's ability to recover from illness and disease. Within
these seven groups, he further identified specific qualities
of what he called temporary 'mood states' and the more
established 'personality types'. He labelled the inclusive nature of these categories as 'Fear, Uncertainty, Insufficient
Interest in Present Circumstances, Loneliness, Over-Sensi-
tivity to Influences and Ideas, Despondency and Despair,
and Over-concern for Welfare of Others'.*

As the work with the remedies progressed over the years,
Bach continued to fine-tune this aspect of his work, including the placement of each of the thirty-eight remedies into
one of the seven categories. This approach emphasized the
heart of his insights on the actual treatment of illness and
disease. His belief was that when faced with illness, each of
us reacts emotionally according to our 'group' mood state
or personality type (the seven categories). We do not react
according to the symptoms of the particular illness or disease. Here again, at the heart of this theory, we find the
number 'seven'.†

Julian Barnard observes that in all likelihood Bach's
working knowledge of the seven-chakra system correspond-
ed to the headings for his mood/personality groups. The
number of these groups, however, was not the only parallel.
Bach concluded there were also 'seven principles' in which a
personality may err in its soul-evolution, a conclusion which
he presented in *Some Fundamental Considerations of Disease and
Cure* (published in 1930). In this work, Bach identifies these
as 'power, intellectual knowledge, love, balance, service, wisdom, and spiritual perfection.'† He later altered his 'seven
principles' into 'the 'seven' beautiful stages of healing: 'love,

*Weeks, DISCOVERIES, pp 39-40
†Barnard, 2002, p. 281

wisdom, certainty, faith, joy, hope and peace'.*

As noted earlier, Bach intended his system of healing to be one of simplicity; but certainly there is a contradiction between this desire and the nature of Bach himself. In reading what little is available of his own writings, it's clear that he was constantly fine-tuning his theories of application, while remaining steadfast in his approach to all things spiritual. As such, his methodology and thought processes are sometimes confusing and sometimes too intellectual.

It appears that when he was speaking of mood states and personality types in the context of his seven groups, he was addressing issues of methodology for treating illness. It's apparent that he didn't intend this approach in treating illness be confused with his earlier writings on soul lessons and the karmic law of rebirth regarding the Twelve Healers as soul types. To re-emphasize a point made earlier, he worked simultaneously on both the mundane and spiritual planes with his remedies. Still, it's not always easy to be certain of Bach's internal thought processes or which 'personal lens' he was looking through. Confusion on our part seems to be more about his constant desire to learn and expand upon what he already knew or was 'shown' (a distinction noted in earlier chapters), rather than not being sure of his knowledge. Despite the frequent amendments to his observations of human nature, it seems that in his mind, there were connections between the traditional characteristics of each major chakra, personality, or mood type, and stages of healing.

In 1934, when Bach settled at Mt Vernon for the final two years of his life, he had identified the twelve soul types, the Twelve Healers, and the Seven Helpers.† Although he

---

*Barnard, COLLECTED WRITINGS, p.101

†The Seven Helpers are Olive, Gorse, Oak, Vine, Heather, Rock Water and Wild Oat

believed his work was now complete, this was not to be. During 1935, he discovered what we know today as the final nineteen remedies. These were the remedies he considered 'more spiritualized', functioning at a higher vibration than the original 'twelve' soul type remedies or the additional 'seven helpers'.*

The significance of these additional nineteen is that they relate to emotional responses we may have to 'in the moment' events. However, these events, although current, can fire reactions tied to our personal history through our subconscious memories. Even though we aren't conscious of these connections, our deep subconscious bond to the subtle familiarity of past experiences creates an instant awareness that manifests the same fears, insecurity, apathy, guilt, or shame. Often these are referred to as 'hot buttons' or 'knee-jerk reactions'. The bad news is that we're so comfortable with these responses that we aren't aware of our unhealthy history with them. Once again, as a tool in our toolbox, the Moon's nodal patterns in our astrological birth chart provide clues as to why we have this unhealthy history and how, with the help of the remedies, we can switch the channel.

As Bach was also a homeopath, we can see the parallels here to homeopathic philosophy in his approach to these final nineteen remedies and the spiritual axiom 'as above, so below', found in homeopathic theory. Considered vibrational or energy medicine, homeopathic theory views the higher vibrations or potency of certain remedies as possessing the ability to heal us at deeper levels. In Bach's observation, with the final nineteen remedies functioning at a 'higher vibration', he was also saying that their efficacy could balance out deep, toxic emotions.

From an energetic perspective, the emotional patterns

*Barnard, COLLECTED WRITINGS, p. 23

of our chakras are about as far down as we can excavate – should we wish to go there. More often than not, we try to pass on this, saying to ourselves, I'll negotiate, I'll do anything but *that*; it isn't so bad. The conflict here is that our soul is trying to push us for our own good, but as humans, we're internally wired to resist this effort. While we consciously believe that we're 'in charge', our resistance plays out through repetitive, toxic history. Unaware that our soul's will is far wiser and more powerful, our resistance eventually brings us to our knees either physically or metaphorically – sometimes both. As we teeter on the edge of our personal abyss, we ask ourselves in wonderment, 'How the blazes did I get here?'

This is the moment when we need to take an inventory of our chakras, their emotional patterns, and our participation in how we 'got here'. Fortunately, we have tools to work with, our twelve soul types, the seven helpers, and the final nineteen remedies. This is when we can take the plunge with our karmic and current emotional baggage, and head further along on our evolutionary journey.

[These] beautiful remedies, which have been Divinely enriched with healing powers ... open up those channels to limit more light of the Soul, that [we] may be flooded with healing virtue.... The action of these remedies is to raise our vibrations and open up our channels for the reception of our Spiritual Self, to flood our natures with the particular virtue we need.... They cure, not by attacking disease, but by flooding our bodies with the beautiful vibrations of our Higher Nature, in the presence of which disease melts as snow in the sunshine. *

*Barnard, COLLECTED WRITINGS, p. 117

FOURTEEN

It's All in the Chakras

*'Chakras are organizational centers for the reception,
assimilation, and transmission of life force energy. They are
the stepping stones between heaven and earth.'*
Anodea Judith

WHETHER WE respond to our environment
with faith or fear depends in large part upon
the emotional and energetic patterns rooted in
our chakras. These patterns, when expanded, bring us into
a state of authentic balance, wellbeing and faith. As we've
seen previously, we incarnate into this lifetime with karma
to burn off, and as we work on this, our chakra patterns
typically fluctuate between contraction and expansion. This
fluctuation is part of the process through which we heal old
emotional wounds and at the same time create new ones.
Unfortunately, one of the difficulties we encounter is that
for most of us it usually takes a physical malfunction for the
problem to get our attention.

Western medicine would have us believe that the true
nature of being 'healed' is manifested by the absence of disease. From a spiritual point of view, and certainly from Edward Bach's perspective, healing goes far deeper than our
physical, cellular, self. True healing is the transformation not
only of body but also of mind and emotions, down into the
depths of our spirit. This is a goal we're compelled to work
toward, one fuelled by our soul's intent that we connect to

its purpose through the purification fires of our feelings and emotional process.

In the previous chapter, I set out the seven stages of healing Bach identified: *peace, hope, joy, faith, certainty, wisdom and love,* in that order. But, if we consider these stages in a different order, as they relate to the traditional themes of the seven chakras, a very interesting scenario takes shape. Additionally, if we consider the relationship between the final nineteen remedies (i.e., those identifying emotions 're-actionary' to our environment), the seven steps of healing and the seven chakras, we're presented with an opportunity that can help us progress further along our mystical path.

While Bach believed the final nineteen remedies were more spiritualized and functioned at a higher vibration, it's important to remember that they're no more important than the first nineteen. However, although there are considerable combinations of Dr Bach's thirty-eight remedies, the final nineteen are particularly valuable tools in our exploration of the emotional patterns lodged in our chakras. While each of the remedies meets us where we are, helping us to get where we need to be, the connection between emotional discord and physical imbalance is a prevailing theme that appears throughout Bach's writings. In HEAL THYSELF, he states:

> *It cannot be too firmly realized that every soul in incarnation is down here for the specific purpose of gaining experience and understanding, and of perfecting his personality towards those ideals laid down by the soul. No matter what our relationship be to each other, whether husband and wife, parent and child, brother and sister, or master and man, we sin against our Creator and against our fellowmen if we hinder from motives of personal desire the evolution of another soul. Our sole duty is to obey the dictates of our own conscience.... Let everyone remember that his Soul has laid*

down for him a particular work, and that unless he does this work, though perhaps not consciously, he will inevitably raise a conflict between his Soul and personality which of necessity reacts in the form of physical disorders. *

In this statement, although somewhat lengthy, Bach was quite clear about potential outcomes for anyone who chooses to ignore their soul's agenda. For those of us in pursuit of discovering our soul's purpose on our journey, contraction and imbalance are obstacles to moving forward. Here, the importance of attaining a sense of emotional wellbeing cannot be overstated. Unfortunately, we're not always able to take an 'objective pulse' of where contracted emotional patterns show up in our chakras. Sometimes we're in such a state of emotional discord we can't even see where we are, much less conjure up the ability to make a connection between the problem and the remedies we need.

Back in Chapter Two, I discussed Caroline Myss' well-known expression, 'your biography is your biology'. Just as this core tenet of holistic healing was put forward by Dr Bach nearly a century ago, in so many words, the truth in them remains in Myss' contemporary vocabulary; when an internal, emotional imbalance isn't addressed, the body at some point won't be able to maintain the stress and will break down.

In exploring the state of the emotional patterns of our chakras, Myss' statement points the way to a very important map for us. In the genuine sense of holistic healing, there's never a single solution, as there are many parts to the whole. For example, we can attain a greater sense of self-awareness through our feelings and emotions, but we also can look to physical clues from our body. For some, paying attention to

*Barnard, COLLECTED WRITINGS, p. 140

physical clues may be a more obvious pathway to recognizing there are imbalances in their chakras. The expression, 'listen to your body', isn't an idle one. By being able to identify 'where it hurts', we have clues as to where we're stuck through the emotional and physical themes of each of the chakras. Once we can identify our 'contracted theme(s)', we can turn to the remedies to assist us in moving from a vulnerable emotional state to an expansive state.

Published some years ago now, Myss' message in ANATOMY OF THE SPIRIT (1996) and WHY PEOPLE DON'T HEAL AND HOW THEY CAN (1997), that both emotional and physical issues can manifest for each chakra, still holds true. Myss' scheme appears in abbreviated format as follows.

Chakra	Organs	Mental/Emotional Issues	Physical Dysfunctions
First	Base of spine, immune system	Family and group safety/secutrity	Depression, chronic lower back pain, immune disorders
Second	Sexual organs, regions up to small intestine	Blame, guilt, creativity, power	Chronic lower back pain, sexual difficulties, sciatica
Third	Abdomen, stomach, regions up to the heart	Trust, self-esteem, sensitivity to criticism	Arthritis, colon/intestinal problems, liver dysfunction
Fourth	Heart, lungs, breasts	Love, hatred, resentment, grief, hope	Cardiac/pulmonary difficulties, allergies, breast cancer
Fifth	Throat, teeth hypothalamus	Personal expression, addiction	Mouth and throat difficulties

Sixth	Brain/nervous system	Truth, self-evaluation, intelligence	Neurological difficulties, seizures, learning difficulties
Seventh	Muscular, skeletal systems	Faith, spirituality, ability to see larger picture	Energetic disorders, extreme sensitivity to environmental factors

In reviewing Myss' interpretations, we may note that she addresses these relationships in the extreme. But clearly, imbalances in these centres can and do exist without manifesting to these edges. Taking these concepts to a much broader and deeper level, a considered and introspective assessment of how specifically contracted and expanded emotional patterns within our chakras influence our mental, physical and spiritual health will be explored in the following chapters. This examination is a necessary part of our personal excavation, because it holds remedy clues from Dr Bach's Final Nineteen as necessary tools in order for us to discover our soul's intended purpose toward evolutionary growth. By paying attention to our emotions, along with suggested remedy solutions, we can find support in our quest toward chakra expansion and interconnected harmony.

FIFTEEN

Taking Root: the First Chakra

Walnut & Cherry Plum – Hope

Return to the root and you'll find the meaning
Sengcan (Zen Patriarch, Sixth Century)

A S IN ALL THINGS of an esoteric nature, there are subtle differences between interpretations, but it's generally accepted that the 'physical' locations of our first six chakras are represented by two triangles, one with a broad base and the point above and the other an inversion of this, forming the spiritually significant six-pointed star. In this imagery, the root, sacral, and solar plexus chakras exist in the lower triangle. Our diaphragm (the organ in our body responsible for regulating our breathing), is the physiological separation between these chakras, with the upper triangle symbolizing the heart, throat and brow chakras. The crown or seventh chakra is nonphysical as it's located above the crown of the head. Some spiritual teachings inform us that the emotional chakra patterns of the lower triangle play out through relationships of our physical life, while those of the upper triangle are more concerned with our spiritual awakening.* As we continue on our journey, it's important to keep in mind that the emotional patterns and imprints within each chakra influence our relationships. Regardless of whether they're in a state of contraction or expansion, the state of our chakras influenc-

*Hodgson, THE STARS AND THE CHAKRAS, p. 75

es our relationships physically, emotionally and spiritually.

According to schools of eastern philosophical thought, our so-called first chakra is located at the base of the spine. This chakra is where we take root, so to speak; it's in the place which grounds us to the earth. Foundations are exceedingly important in our lives, because in form and function they're the underpinnings of the structures and environments in which we live and work. In our body, our feet and legs provide our foundational support for the physical core in which we live. If the foundations that support us in a physical, philosophical, and energetic sense are unstable, we are indeed on very shaky ground.

From both energetic and psychological perspectives, the first chakra is where we connect to our tribe or family identity. This chakra is also the reference and anchor to our determination in this life. In the grander scheme of things, when this chakra is in an expanded state, we're acutely aware of the Divine Universe and our connection to it. Unfortunately, achieving this connection is difficult. Still, we continue to pursue our sacred shopping in order to do so. Universal connection and brotherhood are the expansive goals of our first chakra and our job is to work toward them.

Conversely, the first chakra is where our belief-systems are challenged. Such challenges bring us face to face with an assortment of conflicts manifesting in emotional chaos and physical difficulties. How does this happen? It happens when we plug into family or tribal agendas that superficially feel appropriate. In reality, these agendas can be, and often are, in conflict with our soul's agenda; something that frequently shows up in a birth chart through the evolutionary astrological lens. The repetitive message in Bach's philosophy, that each of us has a soul job to do in this life, doesn't mean our soul path is going to be accepted with open arms from the rest of our 'earthly family'.

Key issues of this chakra are *survival* and *safety*. Just 'thinking about' these things can often rouse contraction of the chakra – what would happen if I were to 'go against the tide', risking abandonment by my family or tribe? How would I survive? Could I survive? Further, do we feel a threat to our safety in any way? The issues of survival and safety are so basic they create visceral reactions in the body when we perceive threats of any kind. In these instances, threats to our survival and safety can cause this chakra to contract to such an extent that we become incapable of moving forward physically, much less emotionally.

We first met legendary psychologist, Abraham Maslow (1908–1970) in the discussion around a Taurus Moon in our natal chart. Now we meet his famous pyramid of human needs again as our need for safety and security within family and tribe find their natural home in our root chakra and are paramount for us to function and survive in a chaotic world.*

When the first chakra is in a chronic state of contraction, triggered by emotions and feelings of fear for our survival, there is a heavy toll on our immune system, shifting the chemistry in our body. The result is that our immune system eventually deteriorates. This kind of interference in our chemistry can first appear as something mildly bothersome, such as lower back pain (no support there) escalating to psychological depression (from mild to extreme) and/or life-threatening illnesses such as cancer and heart disease.

Once we discover the area of contraction, we can then examine the remedies required to help our expansion. In this case, **Walnut** is:

The Remedy for those who have decided to take a great step forward in life, to break old conventions, to leave old limits and restrictions

*http//web.utk.edu/~gwynne/maslow.htm

and start on a new way… a great spell-breaker, both of things of the past commonly called heredity, and circumstances of the present. *

While Bach considered Walnut the 'right remedy' for protecting us from unwanted outside influences, this wasn't his only consideration in the application of Walnut. As we can see from the above quotation, he also felt one could call upon Walnut to assist us in breaking old patterns and what can be considered 'toxic' ties.

The American author John Bradshaw, noted for his work in interpersonal relationships back in the 1980s and 90s, used the phrase 'the ties that bind' regarding toxic relationships and circumstances in our lives that prevent us from manifesting our highest potential. In terms of our spiritual path, such toxicity stops us from moving towards discovering our soul's purpose.

When the root (first) chakra is in a contracted state, family/tribal relationships by their very nature keep us tethered in unhealthy ways. They keep us so intimately, and sometimes so cunningly, bound that we don't recognize they're the very source of our emotional impotence. This toxic binding can manifest in the co-dependent behaviour discussed in connection to Centaury, in Chapter Eight. Because key issues of the root chakra are safety and survival, severing toxic ties for many seems out of the question. Furthermore, a contracted state of this chakra is a welcome breeding-ground for what the author Julia Cameron, who wrote THE ARTIST'S WAY, calls 'crazymakers'.†

*Chancellor, p. 201

†'Crazymakers' is a perfect description fot the negative indication of Bach's White Chestnut remedy. While this particular remedy will not be discussed in these chapters, readers can refer to complete descriptions in any of the sources on the Bach remedies listed in 'Further Reading'.

According to Cameron, crazymakers 'are those person-alities who create storm centres'. Among their behavioural characteristics she includes their ability to break deals and destroy schedules, discount your reality, spending your time and money in the process. Furthermore, crazymakers ex-pect special treatment and are expert blamers who hate or-der.* They're so clever and believable that their appearance into our lives ultimately sets up an internal dialogue that blocks our ability to move forward.

As we will see further on, crazymakers not only lodge in our root chakra, they are part of our karmic contract. Although it may seem that their sole job is to deter us from discovering our soul's purpose, they actually are an impor-tant part of our growth dynamic. A key here rests in how we respond to them and the situations they create for us. From a karmic perspective, crazymakers are actually in our lives to test our mettle. Their unspoken question to us is, do we want to move forward or take a pass, stay where we are, only to repeat the same script (albeit with a different cast), the next time around?

If we're able to come to the awareness that these ele-ments in our lives are responsible for the contraction of our root chakra and the drain on our personal power, Walnut will help us confidently sever those binding ties that keep us stuck. Walnut, however, is not the only remedy we need to consider in our root chakra first aid kit, and that brings us to **Cherry Plum**.

Cherry Plum was the first remedy of the final nineteen Bach discovered. He described Cherry Plum as the remedy for the mind being overworked, unable to take 'strain'. Fur-thermore, he noted, one is in the 'negative' Cherry Plum state:

*Cameron, THE ARTIST'S WAY, 1992, pp 46-9

*When impulses come upon us to do things, we should not in the ordinary way think about or for one moment consider. The remedy for this comes from the Cherry Plum.... This drives away all the wrong ideas and gives the sufferer mental strength and confidence.**

Each of the remedies has an extreme indication of its negative state and for Cherry Plum, this state is contemplation of suicide. Years ago when I was an active Bach Practitioner, I observed this emotional state in some of my clients, but I also saw the action of this remedy lift the fog of perception from the manifestation of the contracted state.

Essential keys in Cherry Plum issues are those of control and internal struggle. Very often in my presentations on the remedies, I used Cherry Plum as an example of Bach's philosophy concerning conflict between the soul agenda and the personality. In the negative state, the individual's internal struggle typically centres on a clash between external moral pressures (particularly in the family/tribe agendas) and internal emotions.

In these circumstances, they experience the pressures of an environment that emphasizes order and mental rationale over the emotions of the soul's intent and happiness. In the more extreme circumstances, forces within that environment can be abusive both emotionally and physically. We only have to look at the rigid cultural, political and religious frameworks that exist today as examples. Thus, the only avenue of escape open to them is emotional shutdown. External characteristics indicating such a state has occurred include irrational hysteria, temper tantrums, and even psychotic behaviour. Signs of depression are not unusual – such as lack of sleep, hopelessness, or episodic outbursts of rage.

Unable to distinguish between the soul's intent and the

*Barnard, COLLECTED WRITINGS, p. 8

moral expectations placed upon the soul and the personality by others, the person can feel as if they are 'coming apart at the seams'. The vulnerable mood state of Cherry Plum is one that is very much about light and dark, according to Barnard.* Recalling Bach's words that the Cherry Plum remedy 'gives the sufferer mental strength and confidence', we can add it to our toolkit for first-chakra contraction should we 'feel' this is the source of our stagnation.

As with each of the chakras, the ideal approach to taking inventory of 'how we are' is contemplative introspection, such as meditation. If we're not familiar with this method and find it difficult to practise in the beginning, we can always look to the body; listen to what the body is telling us and where. If we're honest with ourselves, the clues will rear up before us like red warning lights. Once we recognize these clues, we can consider solutions and the remedies needed so that we can act upon our solutions with **hope**.

*Barnard, 2003, p. 186

SIXTEEN

—

Personal Best, Choice and Resilience: the Second Chakra

Pine, Crab Apple – Peace

A true shaman keeps no secrets about knowledge that can help and heal. The difficulty is not in keeping knowledge secret, but in getting people to understand and use it.... Widely spread knowledge actually has more potency than secrets locked up and unused.... And the sacredness of knowledge lies not in its reservation for a few, but in its availability to many.... And finally, shamans recognize no hierarchy or authority in matters of the mind; if ever a group of people could be said to follow a system of spiritual democracy, it would be the shamans of the world.
Serge Kahlil King, Ph.D. in URBAN SHAMAN

WHILE SOME would put shamans in the category of mystics, there is a difference. The shaman, as a magician, observes and then acts as an agent of change. The mystic observes. In communities, the shaman is the holistic healer, storyteller, priest, and psychotherapist, to name a few of his or her roles.

Concerning matters of illness and death, shamanism focuses on, and works in, the spiritual realms – as does the mystic. For the shaman, illness is caused by one of three major things. Two of these are loss of power and loss of soul. Loss of power essentially means that the power animal or spirit guardian, protecting the individual from the spiritual plane, is no longer around him or her. This loss of power can manifest as 'chronic depression, chronic suicidal tendencies or chronic illness where a person can't seem to maintain his or her own immune system.'*

Loss of soul, or 'soul loss', to a shamanic healer means that a piece of the person's life force or vitality has escaped into the space of 'non-ordinary reality'. Typically, this fragmentation results from some type of experienced trauma or threat. When fragmentation occurs, the bit of life force in question waits in safety for the shaman to facilitate a reconnection to the body through a healing ritual known as 'soul retrieval'. Further, according to the psychologist and author, Jeanne Achterberg: 'Soul loss is regarded as the gravest diagnosis in [shamanism], being seen as a cause of illness and death. Yet it is not referred to at all in modern Western medical books.† Psychologists call the shamanistic concept of 'fragmentation' by the term 'dissociation'.

Given that Bach had an interest in the beliefs and traditions of other cultures, it's possible he came across the subject of shamanic healing. But whether he studied the fundamentals of shamanism extensively is doubtful.§ However, what is interesting is that in writing about the healing powers of the remedies, Bach continually spoke of their ability to give us courage so that we may realize our divinity; in other words, they empower us. Bach's identification of dissociation or disconnection between the soul and the personality as the fundamental cause of illness might be considered 'soul loss' in shamanic terms.¶ However differ-

*See Sandra Ingerman, MA, 'Medicine for the Earth, Medicine for People, in *Alternative Therapies in Health and Medicine* 9.6 (2003) pp. 77-78

†Cameron, THE VEIN OF GOD, New York 1996, p. 78

§ One of the world's foremost authorities on shamanism, Mercia Eliade, was a contemporary of Bach's, although his first book on shamanism wasn't published until 1951.

¶Barnard, COLLECTED WRITINGS, p. 129

ently it's expressed, Bach's philosophy on illness and healing tracks interesting parallels with the philosophies of the healing traditions in shamanism.

While the majority of us may not adhere to or practise shamanic traditions, understanding the concepts of loss of power (disempowerment) and loss of soul (dissociation) is important. This is because as we continue in our process of emotional excavation, we find that contraction of the second chakra is about loss of our creative power. Depending on the extent of this loss, soul fragmentation may be part of the picture as well. The second chakra is the gateway for our life force and all forms of creativity. Given that life force and the power of our creativity are inexorably linked, we can further consider that any impediment to this union has a powerful impact on any progress we make on our evolutionary path.

Additionally, the health of the second chakra profoundly affects the activity or inactivity of the other chakras. When expanded, this chakra is the vibrant core of emotional and spiritual energy, firing our power of choice. This expansion also provides us with resilience from decisions we've made that play out in every relationship of our lives. When the second chakra is in a state of expansion, we're in full ownership of our creative selves. Conversely, when this chakra contracts, the power of choice is not an option and we're critically disempowered and emotionally disabled. Thus, in our disempowerment, the fear of losing control translates into intense attempts to control our internal and immediate external environment. With a second chakra shut down, we're unable to absorb vital life force from the Divine, leading to stagnation and erratic functioning of the other six centres. Physical difficulties relating to sexual health, or problems with our reproductive organs – such as prostate or ovarian cancer and menopausal difficulties, including fibroid cysts – all point to stagnant-energy issues in this chakra. Chronic issues of the lower back, colon, and hip areas also show second-chakra contraction.

In addition, the second chakra is the unconscious dumping-ground for all of our unresolved fears that have to do with relationships. Myss states that within the diverse symptomology of a malfunctioning second chakra, fear of betrayal and loss are primary issues. These can materialize in a myriad of scenarios involving money, sex, loss of power, control, rape (emotionally and physically) or abandonment, to name a few.* As spirit in body, the fabric of our emotions and feelings is a complex weave. Life in the body is difficult; relationships are hard, and it is here, particularly in our second chakra, that our soul lessons concerning the power of choice and relationships play out energetically and spiritually.

Karmically, each of us carries some history of betrayal. Nevertheless, when betrayal is a major theme for us, particularly in personal relationships, our behaviour can lead to dysfunctional control issues. Internally, we may experience mild to extreme anxiety if we feel we're not in control of the surrounding environment. Externally we can become victims of social phobia – or the more extreme version, agoraphobia. One who experiences the dynamics of these disorders cannot socialize well, and may be unable to do so altogether. For example, agoraphobics can become so emotionally paralyzed that they become prisoners in their own homes. Externally, and at the other end of the spectrum, their internal fear of losing control translates into extreme controlling behaviour that's dictatorial in its interaction with everything and everyone around them. Sadly, this behaviour leads to disconnection from others and possibly

*Myss, ANATOMY, p. 130

disassociation: surely a lonely existence. At the root of the betrayal theme lie emotional issues of guilt, shame, and an internal message of self-deprecation that tells us erroneously we're undeserving of making choices. Clearly, if one is functioning in a state of shame or guilt, there's little hope of capturing or manifesting the soul's desired path.

When we spiral into hypercriticism, the environment around us – including parenting, partnerships, cultural, and religious models that are part of everyday reality – has triggered second chakra issues. As we noted in Chapter Four, the 'holy anorexia' that manifested in medieval nunneries is a perfect example of internal control issues within an extremely controlling religious environment. Within our framework of the remedies, this behaviour is a reactive 'lashing out' of an extreme negative Pine state. Nevertheless, the 'crazymakers' who are part of these landscapes are a 'soul set-up', giving us the opportunity to overcome these obstacles so that we can retrieve the power we're meant to have. If we continually experience outcomes in our relationships wherein others ignore our needs and our dreams are shattered, we feel betrayed.

Because of these feelings, we have a built-in internal warning mechanism that raises 'red flags'. Through these experiences, our soul is sending us a powerful message: Take responsibility'! It's urging us to take a personal inventory and evaluate our contributions to the relationships that continually create disappointing scenarios. With a contracted second chakra, taking an objective inventory is a tough assignment, because this process potentially brings to light the additional self-deprecation and emotional distress we must examine in order to determine how we arrived at this 'place'.

A more obvious approach at this point may be to check in with our physical wellbeing. If we're emotionally or mentally unaware of contracted energy in this chakra, our body certainly has many ways to give us clues. In the Bach repertoire, **Pine** and **Crab Apple** are two remedies with compelling ability to shift our perception from disempowerment to empowerment, even when our choices don't produce the expected outcome.

A constricted emotional Pine state is one that's reflected in shame-based guilt. In this state, one operates from a core of unworthiness, simply by being in the body. From day one in this incarnation, the contracted Pine mood state or personality type feels and believes they are unworthy. They tend to ruminate over what they have done, did not do, should have done or said. Additionally, those stuck in the second chakra, manifesting the constricted Pine state, will often take on the responsibility for another's dysfunction. 'It's my fault' is their chronic internal and external dialogue.

Unfortunately, their repetitive episodes of betrayal reinforce this belief. Because they're laden with shame and guilt, they believe they're always the problem and always the reason behind these episodes. It's doubtful this assessment is accurate, but in their minds, it is – and therefore, they can never do enough or say enough. In a phrase, they will 'never be enough' and this belief leads to additional dysfunctional forms of behaviour.

If we can momentarily set Pine aside, the remedy Crab Apple with its similarities to, and the very subtle differences from, the negative Pine state is worthy of valuable consideration. For Bach, the Crab Apple remedy was the remedy of 'purification'.* Its constricted state in many ways is similar to the constricted Pine state when lodged in the second chakra, in that both have to do with shame and guilt. However, the shame of Crab Apple manifests in the belief of

*Barnard 2002, p. 229

not being internally clean enough. Thus, in this constricted state, there's an intense belief of internal self-disgust.

Evidence of this constricted state in the second chakra usually surfaces through specific issues of cleanliness and sexual dysfunction that can manifest in obsessive behaviour. It's not unusual for someone stuck in the constricted Crab Apple state to become so fixated on some insignificant physical impurity (usually having to do with the skin), that they totally miss a more serious health issue. When the second chakra is constricted and the Crab Apple remedy is indicated, there's an underlying belief held by the person that some poison is present and must be eradicated from the body. The problem is that as long as the constriction remains, the expulsion is never complete. The belief surrounding impurity totally blocks the infusion of spiritual light and creativity into this chakra. Sexually this constriction can manifest in impotence, frigidity or a general belief that sexual enjoyment is 'dirty behaviour' or 'sinful'.

Ironically, the constricted states of both Pine and Crab Apple typically manifest in the drive for perfection and in over-achievement. Examples of extremes in these dynamics are prominent in the behaviours found in people who suffer from eating disorders such as Anorexia Nervosa and Bulimia.*

As I mentioned in earlier chapters, while Bach considered that the Twelve Healers represented soul types and their lessons, he later recognized that these specific remedies also represented personality types and temporary mood states as well. An example of this interconnection between the thirty-eight remedies can be seen in the zealous contraction

---

*Mack, Gaye, 'Exploring Impications of Treating Eating Disorders with Vibrational Medicine as an Integrative Therapy', 1999, DePaul University, Chicago, Illinois

of Vervain and its relationship to the obsessive, controlling behaviour of negative Pine and Crab Apple. As these vulnerable states escalate, in their drive to over-achieve and in their anxiety to control, their subjects further take on the contracted state of Vervain, which can be intensely zealous and fanatical. The difference here is that the root of Vervain is enthusiasm, while the roots of Pine and Crab Apple are guilt and shame. In the negative Pine and Crab-Apple states, the question arising refers to the type of guilt/shame. For those in the contracted Pine state, it's about what they have done; for those in the contracted Crab Apple state, it's about who they are. Frequently, they can and will manifest both negative states simultaneously.

Worth noting, perhaps, is that Bach had a particular relationship to Pine. We know from Nora Weeks that he experienced the vulnerable states of each of the final nineteen remedies just prior to their discovery. Furthermore, we also know from Weeks that Bach worked in his father's foundry for three years with some difficulty, before approaching his father about attending medical school. Weeks reports that behind this delay in expressing his desire to study medicine, was the feeling that he could not ask his parents for the necessary funds required.* Why was this? Barnard speculates that as the oldest son, perhaps Bach thought he should go into the family business. If this were the case, and he was finding it difficult to separate from this expectation, aspects of Walnut (as discussed in Chapter Fifteen) are clear. Here, however, it seems there's more between the lines in Bach's personal history. In HEAL THYSELF, Bach takes issue with the nature of parenting:

> *The whole attitude of parents should be to give the little newcomer*
> *all the spiritual, mental and physical guidance to the utmost of*

*Weeks, DISCOVERIES, pp 12-13

*their ability, ever remembering that the wee one is an individual soul come down to gain his own experience and knowledge in his own way according to the dictates of his Higher Self, and every possible freedom should be given for unhampered development. ***

He later seems to reiterate his beliefs about parenting in FREE THYSELF using a somewhat stronger voice:

So many suppress their real desires and become square pegs in round holes: through the wishes of a parent, a son may become a solicitor, a soldier, a business man, when his true desire is to become carpenter.... This sense of duty is then a false sense of duty, and a dis-service to the world; it results in unhappiness and, probably, the greater part of a lifetime wasted before the mistake can be rectified.†

Clearly, Bach was addressing, in so many words, the second-chakra issue of empowerment through choice; and equally important, our ability to embrace resilience from our choices regardless of the ramifications. Bach himself possessed an intensive drive for completing tasks that in some respects was obsessive. Furthermore, this behaviour and his recurring theme of life and soul path choices indicate that Pine and second chakra issues were significant for him on a deeply personal level. For him, his writings were a vehicle through which he could safely express the dissatisfactions and frustrations that were part of his own personal history. And yet, it's worth recalling the discussion in Chapter Eleven regarding his karmic path as it related to the evolutionary nodal axis in his birth chart. Despite his frustrations, it would seem that at a deep level, Bach was aware of his soul's intention for him in this life and he listened. Here again is a subtle reminder that although he was

*Barnard, COLLECTED WRITINGS, p. 138   †ibid., p. 97

brilliantly gifted and a mystic, Bach, like the rest of us, was challenged by his own personal dragons.

On our own journey, it's important that we examine how we make our choices and the reasons behind making the decisions we do. We need to keep in mind this is a second-chakra issue and that the second chakra is the seat of our creative energy. While the constriction of this chakra impedes the flow of creativity, we can call upon the remedies of Pine and Crab Apple to assist us. As the remedies aid our ability to shift our emotional energy and perspective, we have the opportunity to discover our power of choice and resilient strength. Moreover, with these, we're able to embrace a sense of internal *peace* with our decisions, knowing that we're free to make different choices.

SEVENTEEN

—

Solar Power: the Third Chakra

Larch, Willow & Holly – Joy

'No one can make you feel inferior without your consent'
Eleanor Roosevelt

WITH THE THIRD chakra, we come to the last centre of the lower triangle in our chakra symbology of the triangles. In the 'last but not least' category, its placement is far from insignificant, as we make our way upwards into the upper triangle. Located in what is known as the solar plexus of our body, this chakra is the seat of our internal self-command of our exterior environment. This is where our conscious 'fire' lives. It's the fire we need in order for us to progress forward when faced with karmic challenges along our soul path. As the centre of the normal feelings and emotions, this is where we consciously experience everyday life – through our joys, desires, anger, ambitions, anxieties, and/or fears of failure and success. Finally, this centre represents the alchemical melting pot or union of the expanded authority achievable in our first and second centres.

As I described in Chapters Fifteen and Sixteen, the first and second chakras represent the fostering of healthy ties within the greater collective and the realization that exercising the power of choice is necessary in order to follow our soul's intended path. It's important for us to remember, also, that separation from the 'tribe' or tribal ways is sometimes necessary for us to move forward. Furthermore, in any such separation we're often propelled into activating the power of choice that, as unique souls, we're entitled to.

In Chapter Six, it was put forward that Dr Bach believed each of us has incarnated in this life with a soul lesson to transform. By working to shift the hindrance of our particular lesson into its quality or virtue, we have the opportunity to offer the benefits of its virtue to other human beings. The intensity and harmony of our third-chakra fire depends on how well we have learned to balance the emotional patterns of the tribal male energy of the first chakra and the creative feminine energy of our second chakra. Determining our progress in the expansion of the first two chakras is vital, because this progress has a direct impact on our sense of self and the contributions we can make to the environment around us and the world.

As with each of the chakra centres, formidable challenges face us in this, the third. Third-chakra issues include sensitivity to outward critics, invalidation by others, lack of self-esteem, and the inability to trust our intuitive voice, the voice of our soul. So, we have our work cut out, as we discover that this chakra involves both internal and external development.

In Chapter Five, we met the concept of the 'hungry ghost', described by psychologist, Jack Kornfield. The hungry ghost that lives in each of us is our chronic wanting; if we only had more, we could do more, be more. On our evolutionary path, we discover that our wanting can fuel our solar fire either positively or negatively, and that the third chakra is the battleground of these polarities. The emotional experiences we have with our external and internal environment reflect the degree of success or failure in this challenge. The question becomes, how do these reflections manifest?

We find that the core health of this centre, emotionally, physically, and spiritually, is reflected in the security we experience through our self-esteem, or alternatively in the lack of it. As Caroline Myss observes, 'No one is born with healthy self-esteem. We must earn this quality in the process of living as we face our challenges one at a time.'*

We need to remember then, that on the spiritual level, we attract relationships and circumstances that give us opportunities to transform contracted states of our chakras into states of expansion. When our third centre is contracted, our self-esteem is weak – and for some of us totally non-existent. In this state, there's a lack of self-confidence as well as a lack of the ability to succeed in the external world. We're unaware that we're compromised, because we easily defer to others – believing they are smarter, more experienced, have more talent, and are more creative. In a simple phrase, *they are more and we are invisible.* In our deferment, we've abdicated not only our personal power but also our divinity.

Still, deferment isn't the only manifestation of a weakened self-esteem. Just as easily as we defer, we can also go on the attack, full of fiery acrimonious energy. This energy can fuel attitudes and actions of arrogance, intimidation, self-righteousness, and abusive anger; or we can simply be obnoxiously opinionated. Regardless of which of the many exterior expressions our weakened self-esteem takes, they're always about dumping our toxic emotions on others. They all mask a gut fear of 'not being' and a fear that we're fated to be swallowed up by our environment.

In addition, third-chakra contraction prevents access to our intuition and blocks 'soul messages' from coming through. It skews our perceptions. Through the lens of our hypersensitivity, we misinterpret innocuous remarks

*ANATOMY, p. 169

and behaviour by others. Constructive observations, suggestions, even innocent humour and conduct all translate as criticism intended to spotlight our self-assigned lack of intelligence and abilities. Thus, feeling invalidated by the external world, we protect our secret of low or non-existent self-esteem through misguided reactions.

Contracted, the fire of the third chakra fans the flames of rage and anger shrouded in verbal lashings or recriminations spewed out toward others. In more extreme reactions, physical vindictiveness may emerge. In any case, all of these responses are smokescreens for the shame of inadequacy. Further, such behaviour carries a double-edged sword. At the very least, it most certainly hurts those who become targets. And it carries the potential of relationships being severed altogether. Leaving behind a trail of relationship ashes, we move from one encounter to the next, never clearly understanding 'what happened'. The irony is that those whom we respond to most negatively, whether it be with arrogance, intimidation, self-righteousness or abuse, are the very people our soul has chosen to help us strengthen our self-esteem and value.

Energetically, the third chakra centre is where we assimilate either healthy or unhealthy energy from our environment. It's also where we may 'leak' the energy needed to discover our soul's intended purpose for us and how to manifest it. We are spirit in body, but from the physical perspective the impact of third-chakra contraction is enormous. As the solar plexus is the gravitational centre of our physicality, imbalance in this centre is a tenuous two-way street. Physical manifestations include difficulties with the upper intestine, abdominal area, liver, gallbladder, adrenals, spleen and mid spine.*

*ANATOMY, p. 96

From an Ayurvedic perspective:*

The intestinal tract is at the centre of the organizational plan that governs human functions. It is the crux of the matter. This notion is echoed in other traditions, too.... There seems to be a sort of consensus that it is here where health is rooted and where disease originates.†

To Ayurvedic and other holistic practitioners, the state of our emotions is a vital variable in the overall picture of our harmony. If our emotions are not at peace, particularly in the third chakra, we can easily move into a state of dysbiosis (disorder in the intestinal tract). As a bacteriologist, Edward Bach repeatedly wrote about the necessity of intestinal cleanliness.§ Perhaps it was from examining the philosophies of the East that he came to subscribe to this belief. However, it's not only our intestinal health at risk when our third centre is contracted. It's often said that the liver is the seat of unresolved anger that smoulders, and that we 'vent' anger through our spleen. Furthermore, negative emotions drain energy from our adrenals. Overall, any of these unhealthy conditions are catalysts for a depleted immune system. Whether we regain or do not regain vigorous health may depend on the severity of this downward spiral. Unfortunately, from the spiritual plane, when we ignore soul signals and messages, once again, the Divine will bring us to our knees through the only vehicle we seem to understand at this point – our body. This begs the question, how many times do we need to hear this message?

It's important to make mention here of an attitude that cropped up in many new-age circles back in the 1980s and onward. Among the toxic shame-based tenets of this

*Ayurveda is the ancient ssystem of holistic medicine originating in India.   †Ballantine, p. 249   §Barnard, 2002, p. 229

movement was the philosophy advocating illness and disease as punishment foisted upon us by 'spirit'. This punitive belief was, and is, in direct contrast to Bach's beliefs and writings:

> *It matters not our stage of advancement, whether aborigine or disciple, this is of no consequence as regards health; but what is important is that we, whatever our station, live in harmony with the dictates of our soul.... During our sojourn in search of perfection, there are various stages… and we have to master stage by stage as we progress. Some stages may be comparatively easy, some exceedingly difficult, and then it is that disease occurs, because it is at those times that we fail to follow our Spiritual Self, that the conflict arises which produces illness.* *

Thus, according to Bach, illness isn't a matter of punishment, but a matter of notification that we're not 'listening'.

Recalling that the different permutations of the thirty-eight remedies are several, various aspects of each remedy are effective in addressing forms of third-chakra contraction. As an example, we can also consider Pine and Crab Apple – discussed in the last chapter in connection with the 'shame' aspect found in this centre. Additionally, practitioners traditionally use Walnut to help protect and seal the solar plexus from unwanted energy assimilation and drain. And there are three other remedies particularly useful for the maladies experienced from contraction in this centre.

Larch is the remedy Bach identified for issues of self-esteem. As lack of self-esteem is the core emotion driving contraction in our third centre, Larch is extremely important. Recalling Myss' statement that self-esteem is not something we are born with, but something that we must earn, a contracted third chakra is mirrored by the negative Larch state and one that results from life and/or relationship difficul-

*Barnard, COLLECTED WRITINGS, p. 158

ties. Similar to Pine and Crab Apple, negative Larch can be the result of an individual having to endure years of harsh criticism, belittlement, or lack of encouragement and support. This leaves little desire to extend to the outside world, as the internal belief is that failure is a probable outcome, no matter what is attempted. Someone in the extreme state of lacking self-confidence won't even try because they know they'll fail.

Larch as a remedy in one's formula* works to bolster self-confidence by shifting the perception into one that aids in understanding that each of us is blessed with divine gifts that are unique and meant to be contributed to benefit those around us. While self-confidence is the core issue in third-chakra contraction, we also need remedies to help shift the negative behaviour through which we express this shame.

As noted earlier, smouldering, unresolved anger can be deadly to us on a physical level, especially in matters involving the liver. This makes sense since the liver is the organ responsible for detoxifying our body. The holistic author, Louise Hay, identifies cancer in general as the manifestation of long-held resentment eating away at us internally.† From a chakra perspective, we're reminded by both of the authors I have mentioned – Myss and Hay – that holistic philosophy identifies unresolved emotional issues 'stuck' in a particular chakra through the physical location of illness points. According to Dr Bach, the remedy needed for resentment, bitterness and/or self-pity is **Willow**. In the negative emotional state, the Willow mood§ can exhibit any or all of these particular emotions. Typically, those in this state

---

*Refer to 'Practical Matters' at the end of this book for information on creating a 'personal remedy formula'   †Hay, p. 12

§Interestingly, Bach did not identify Willow as also being a personality type

point the finger of blame at everyone and everything else as being the source of their problems. The subtle message behind this state is that the person never 'owns' their participation or non-participation in their situation. This contraction is most likely a carry-over from issues of shame and guilt in the second chakra, thus compounding the situation. Unable to access the energy needed to transform their compromised self-esteem, they simply cannot get to the place where they understand that in taking some degree of responsibility for their actions they're on their way to building up their struggling self-esteem.

Several years ago, a psychotherapist and I shared a client who was in a negative Willow state. Working as a part-time nurse, with two children under the age of five and a husband who travelled constantly, she was someone who clearly had a lot on her plate. Over the course of many months, the therapist and I worked with various remedy-combinations to help this woman with the obsessive-compulsive behaviours she was using as a form of self-medication. *

On the surface, the client never verbally expressed resentment of her situation or blame; in fact, it was quite the opposite. Raised in the strict Catholic tradition, she bore her situation with an air that sometimes resembled martyrdom. However, it wasn't until she became pregnant with her third child that she lamented the situation in which she had obviously taken part, at which point I realized I was seeing negative Willow. I stopped her current formula and suggested Willow by itself. Being very compliant, the client began taking

*Bach believed the process of harmonizing our emotions required not just one remedy, but often a combination of remedies. As such, the combination an individual might begin with changes as the emotions shift in their harmonization. This process is often referred to in practice as a 'peeling of the onion'.

Willow immediately and within forty-eight hours was on the phone to her therapist crying in the realization that 'she had been setting [herself] up for self-sabotage all of these years'.

It's interesting to note that the negative Willow state has an aspect of inflexibility or resistance about it, through the refusal to take responsibility for oneself. Conversely, the remedy brings flexibility to the person through the willingness to participate in his/her process and the awareness of how this process fits into the overall picture of his/her intended soul growth. It's also important to note that it's rare for the remedies to work so quickly when deep-seated issues are involved. Here, however, it's likely that subconsciously her misery was so intense that she was at a point where she was ready to participate in her 'excavation' at a deeper level. Thus, the Willow acted as a catalyst in bringing her to the awareness that *her own* actions were significantly behind her misery. With the help of her therapist and additional formula-combinations, she was ready to address the issues of shame and disempowerment lodged in her second chakra as well.

As I noted earlier, the destructive emotions of anger and rage are not always repressed. We can see, unfortunately, an explosion of these unrepressed emotions being expressed around the globe: this all-too-prevalent 'in your face' rage. However, the reality is that this type of outward expression of rage is a camouflage for compromised self-esteem in this chakra. It's critical to remember that this manifestation of anger is abusive and an indication that the remedy **Holly** is necessary. As a personality or mood state, Bach placed the Holly type in his category, Over-Sensitive to Influences and Ideas. The behaviour of a negative Holly state is very serious because it's mirrored in all forms of abuse. Whether it comes out emotionally or physically, the Holly state is fierce; it's simply a matter of degree. In the extreme contraction, this state is vindictive, hell-bent on revenge. The irony is that this 'personality' is actually very sensitive and has suffered some form of abuse in this life, past lives or both. This reinforces what psychologists know from experience: 'the abuser has been the abused'. Thus, lacking the experience of love, with little or no self-esteem, the negative Holly state 'keeps score' of each perceived cruelty experienced. Internally there's an intense, unhealthy 'burning' that can drive them to lose control, spiralling into a protective behavioural mode of 'payback'. Bach established that individuals exhibiting the negative Holly state or personality type suffer a great deal internally 'often when there is no real cause for their unhappiness'.*

In this observation of Bach's we are again informed that negative emotions have an effect upon our perceptions. To re-emphasize this: when we experience the energy of negative emotions, this experience fuels contraction in our chakras. At the same time, perceptions of our environment become skewed and highly inaccurate. The action of the remedies helps shift these perceptions from unreality to the surrounding reality. Because of their own history of abuse, whether it be emotional, physical or both, someone in this negative state believes everyone is 'out to get them'. This state can only escalate unless they call upon tools to help neutralize their illusions. If this situation is chronic, it's an indication that the person is carrying baggage of a very difficult history and, typically, in need of some type of psychotherapy. With therapeutic assistance and with the help of the remedy Holly (and others), their sensitivities become more balanced, moving into reality. Through this process, those who have had to struggle can now step back and view their experience through a clearer and more realistic lens. Si-

*Barnard, COLLECTED WRITINGS, p.42

multaneously, the third chakra begins to expand, self-esteem builds, and awareness of their soul's intended path becomes their reality and their joy in being engaged in the world.

We now move into the upper triangle of our chakra symbology, beginning with the Fourth Chakra, that of the Heart. It's important to re-emphasize that working with the contracted states of the first three chakra centres is vital if we intend to engage fully on our evolutionary journey. As Caroline Myss states:

> not only do we want to 'know about'... reincarnation, meditation, and spiritual ecstasy, we want to 'live' them. We want the power of these spiritual teachings to activate our biological tissue; we want to feel the presence of God in our bodies as well as in our minds. We want physical contact with the Divine, matching the level of contact previously enjoyed by saints and mystics of the great traditions. *

In order to reach this goal, we first need to 'chop wood, carry water'. In other words, we need to work at the mundane, everyday chores that keep us going and aren't necessarily glamorous. This means showing up, paying attention to what's going on within us at ground level, and excavating toxic emotions. These are necessary keys to the experience of joy. And they are necessary before we can ascend into the ethers.

*Myss, WHY PEOPLE DON'T HEAL, pp 86-87

EIGHTEEN

—

At the Crossroads: State of the Heart, the Fourth Chakra

Beech, Honeysuckle, Star of Bethlehem – Unconditional Love

In Egyptian mythology, there is the general myth that upon death, an individual's heart was weighed by Anubis against the goddess Maat's feather. If the heart was heavy because of foul thoughts and actions, it would outweigh the feather, and the soul would be fed to the shadow world. But if the scales were balanced, showing that the heart of the deceased was pure in intent and that the individual had been just and honourable in life, he would be welcomed by the god Osiris and passage into the sacred land offered.

BACK IN Chapter Two, we began the exploration of our soul's intended evolutionary path. Along the way, we've investigated the five karmic laws, looked into the question of what makes a mystic and come face to face with the emotional dragons that have the power to keep us emotionally 'stuck'. While these hindrances and dragons may intimidate us, we explored the channels of expansion and growth possible with the help of several of the remedies before diving into the 'heart of our story' through the lens of Evolutionary Astrology. And now we now find ourselves faced with a decision.

Even if we've been able to face the work necessary to transform the dragons of the lower centres and the unre-

solved emotions in our nodal karmic story, the question before us is, do we have the actual courage to do the work
required for expansion in the lower three chakras? The answer to this is the key to the quality of our process. The
emotional patterns of these chakras are of the mundane
world. If we're able to shift their contracted configurations,
we have a precious opportunity to journey from the mundane to the wisdom of our spiritual heart and the wisdom
of, in Bach's words, 'the Lord Buddha and other great Masters, who have come down from time to time upon earth to
point out to men [and women] the way to attain perfection'.
First, however, we must decide which emotional pattern will
be the model for our progress. Will it be the consciousness
of constriction held in our lower three chakras, or will it be
consciousness of expansion?

This dilemma returns us to our spot where we started
our journey in Chapter Two: are we willing to take up the
challenges presented by our karmic baggage in order to discover our soul's evolutionary purpose? While we may have
realized the work necessary for our soul growth, we tend to
hear a small voice that says to us, 'Maybe next time; if I stay
put, I don't have to commit to doing any new emotional
work'. Here, one more time, we come face to face with our
internal crazymaker and the recurring theme of choice.

As I've made clear in previous chapters, our soul has
mapped out an agenda for us when we incarnate into this
life. Contained within this agenda is the challenge for us
to love unconditionally. As we study the beginning of the
upper triangle of our chakra symbology, much to our surprise, we find that working with our emotions is essential for
our forward movement, with the heart being the gatekeeper. Thus, we have come to the heart of what matters; it is
this fourth chakra that represents our balance between body

(below) and spirit (above). In other words, 'Heart' matters in all things physical, emotional, and spiritual.

Physically, our heart keeps us alive in the body, for when our heart fails, our body fails. As we learned earlier, through the astrological lens our emotional heart is represented by our natal Moon and the seat of our innate wisdom. It's also our spiritual anchor and record-keeper. However, access to this chakra centre isn't easy, and is often a struggle to obtain.

The heart chakra's vibrant emotional and spiritual energy of unconditional love holds the space for us as we experience the baptism of the four elements through the emotional dragons discussed in Chapter Five. As our record-keeper, it holds the remembrances of the joys, pleasures, and moments of happiness we experience. But it also holds the records of the sorrows, hurts and grievances that can catapult us right back down into the contraction of those dragons dwelling in the lower three chakras. The choice is ours as to where we are going to 'live'.

We must keep in mind that no matter how much sacred shopping we have done and are still doing, in order to be on our genuine mystic path, we must make our way into the heart chakra from the lower three chakras. We don't just decide, 'Oh, ok, if I think about loving unconditionally, I am living it; I don't need to deal with all of that unpleasant emotional stuff'. The temptation to intellectualize our work is, without a doubt, the 'Venus Flytrap' on our mystical path.*

The caveat on our journey is that no matter how hard we try to use the intellectual route to become 'spiritual', it will not work. Energetically and emotionally, access to the

---

*In botany, 'the leaves of Venus Flytrap open wide and on them are short, stiff hairs called trigger or sensitive hairs. When anyone touches these hairs enough to bend them, the two lobes of the leaves snap shut, trapping whatever is inside' (www.botany.org)

heart wisdom is proportional to the expanded or contracted state of each of the lower chakras. As these centres come into balance, the heart expands, supporting the ongoing growth of the upper chakras. The heart centre is 'the centre where we learn to harmonize all the conflicting elements in our nature – all conflicts of mind or emotion'.* It's where we're learning the lesson of the Aquarian Age, the lesson of universal brotherhood; and it's a lesson that is *felt*, not thought about. As the gatekeeper, this chakra is affected by the state of the others. Conversely, *its* emotional state affects the health upon these centres 'below' and 'above'. As in the image of Mercury's fluidity referred to in Chapter Thirteen, there's an ongoing flow of energy upwards and downwards, expansive and contractive.

The expression, 'when your heart speaks, take good notes', is wise advice, for to do otherwise will result in emotional and physical dyspepsia. When contracted, the heart chakra is the unconscious dumping ground for the toxic emotions stuck in the lower three: anger, rage, distrust, loneliness, hatred, resentment and bitterness, to name just a few.

There are volumes written on the dysfunctional ramifications of this particular chakra, but at the source of all difficult emotions lies grief. The experience of grief tells us something has been lost. From the spiritual perspective, our primary grief is in our original separation from Divinity. Thus, the humanness of this emotion with which we struggle is part of the necessary process in reconnecting to our Divinity, or to our higher self. Grief is always a challenge, but what's difficult for us to grasp is that it's part of our expansion process. The psychiatrist Carl Jung believed we should embrace our grief because by doing so, our soul will grow. When we're 'in grief', we're in an intensely painful

*Hodgson, THE STARS AND THE CHAKRAS, p. 134

process; we are *in it* as a therapist friend of mine says. Moreover, it's a state that feels so constricted we cannot imagine we'll ever come through it to the other side. However, the only way out is through. In order to move forward on our mystic path, we must be willing to acknowledge our grief and then be willing to let it go honestly, rather than hang onto it as an excuse for not manifesting our intended soul's purpose. As a powerful messenger, grief tells us, yes, there is loss. But, if we honour the process and move through it, its spiritual message reminds us that the universe waits with an abundance of new possibilities and opportunities for us, and then there is *expansion!*

The manifestations of emotions connected to the grieving process are powerful and can easily lead to physical fallout. Staying 'stuck' in our grief commands a high price, both emotionally and physically. Myss identifies heart-chakra malfunctions as any physical manifestations affecting the lungs, breasts, diaphragm, and of course, the heart itself. Congestive heart failure, heart attacks, allergies, pneumonia, bronchitis, and breast cancer,* all point to contractions of this chakra as do the emotional expressions, 'heartless', 'heart-sick', and 'heartbroken'.

If we refer to Chapters Sixteen and Seventeen, wherein we looked at the emotional profiles and remedy characteristics of Pine, Crab Apple, Willow, Holly and Larch, we can see that the healing dynamics of these remedies can also be considered for working with heart-chakra issues. While this consideration once again shows the adaptability of Dr Bach's thirty-eight remedies, we can explore two additional remedies at this point.

In past lectures, when I spoke about the remedy Beech, I described the emotional contraction of the **Beech** personal-

*Myss, ANATOMY, p. 98

ity or mood state by using the phrase, 'beech bitches', which is the American vernacular that uses 'bitch' as a verb. True to form, this personality type or mood state does just this; it 'bitches'. In this state, the Beech personality sees an external environment that's inexcusably imperfect. For them their experience of the external environment is the unreality of the reality. Their view through such a distorted lens generates behaviour that's judgmental, intolerant, and highly critical of everyone and everything around them – and they keep score of every infraction they perceive directed toward them, in a way similar to constricted Holly.

Their way of being becomes so narrow that they create their own constrictions in the way they function in life and in their relationships with others. Seeking exactness and perfection of others in unrealistic ways, they invite the self-destructive dynamic of isolation into their lives. 'If only the world and everyone in it would adhere to the way it should be', is the negative Beech mantra. Here again are clues to constricted third-chakra issues as well. Simply, if we believe we do not possess self-worth, it's impossible for us to honour the worth in others; the shame is too great, or we just don't see the worth in others.

Because of its inability to lessen the perception of flaws, instead of recognizing what is glorious, this narrow way of being can only affect the state of the heart with an eventual outcome of illness. In cardiac health, it's interesting to consider the parallel between a narrow way of being and a narrowing of the arteries, which in turn constricts the flow of the blood: the carrier of our life's vitality on the physical level.

The positive energy or the vibrations of the remedy Beech, however, act as catalysts, assisting the transformation of their vision. Beech shifts the contracted perception of judgment and intolerance to one that supports the expansion of the heart chakra and thus, expansion of the lower centres. Again, it's important to keep in mind that on our mystic path, everything is interconnected; what affects one chakra, affects them all. Finally, Bach's philosophy on negative Beech was this:

> *It is obvious that none of us is in a position to judge or criticize, for the wisest of us sees and knows only the minutest fragment of the Great Scheme of all things, and we cannot judge, knowing so little, how the Great Plan will work.* *

As I stated earlier in this chapter, although the emotion of grief is a difficult one, it's a necessary part of our incarnated life and our human process in soul growth. Grief is the emotion that teaches us to feel. This doesn't mean we're naturally comfortable with this lesson. Most of us are not. Further, we do not always know that we are in grief or that we are grieving. The state of grieving most familiar to us is the intense sadness that overwhelms us at a time of loss, repeatedly telling others and ourselves that we are 'grieving'. However, being 'in grief' is a much longer process altogether. As an example, one who is 'in grief' may not be aware that they are in grief. The manifestation of behaviours such as anger, rage, and mild to extreme depression, eating disorders, and sexual dysfunction or sleep disorders, can indicate the state of grief besides the sadness we connect with grief. Even if we're not able to identify these emotions as part of this process, we know that at some level we hurt, deeply.

While there are several remedies within the thirty-eight well suited to working with aspects of grief, two are of particular note: **Honeysuckle** and **Star of Bethlehem**.

Traditionally, practitioners consider Honeysuckle for the state of mind in which an individual cannot let go of

*Chancellor, p. 46

the past. Instead, they may long for it (which is a form of grieving) or for someone who has passed over, recalling only pleasant memories, far more comforting than they actually were, or their present reality. This mood state becomes particularly common as we age. Statements such as 'I remember when we....', 'Things were so much better back then', 'I don't know what has happened to the world, it was never like this' are all indications of negative Honeysuckle.

However, there is another hue to this mood, and it has to do with emotional wounding and the grief it creates. Some years ago, I had a psychotherapist tell me that, in her opinion, emotional wounds went far deeper than physical wounds. She went on to say that physical wounds could heal; often the emotional wounds stay with us for this lifetime and into the next. As we have also seen through the evolutionary astrological lens, we carry our emotional wounds from past lifetimes into this one.

Earlier, I mentioned the term Caroline Myss uses for the attitude that keeps us stuck in our history, 'woundology'. She says, 'I have ... become convinced that when we define ourselves by our wounds, we burden and lose our physical and spiritual energy and open ourselves to the risk of illness'.*. In our 'woundology', we struggle with the emotional wounds embedded in our past. While we may not be aware of the wounding that drives the contraction of the lower chakras, as discussed up to this point, we're very aware of emotional wounds that have hit us, like the proverbial arrow, right in the heart. Relationship wounds stemming from our 'family of origin' and other relationship difficulties fit into Myss' account of woundology. But we can experience emotional wounding from other sources as well, such as those tied to the disappointment of unrealized

*Myss, WHY PEOPLE DON'T HEAL, p. 6

expectations. While we may only be aware of our wounding to some degree (usually cloaked in situational memories), we know someone or something has hurt us and the memories play like a broken record. They may indeed play so continually that in our grief, we find it difficult to let go and move on. In the contracted Honeysuckle state, we don't expect any happiness, ever.

As a remedy, Honeysuckle in some ways works like Walnut. Recalling that Walnut assists us in breaking the ties we need to break in order to move on, Honeysuckle helps to bring us into the present so that we can take advantage of all it has to offer us. Then, as a result of the Honeysuckle process, we have the opportunity to move forward as our soul intended. Bach described Honeysuckle as the 'Remedy to remove from the mind the regrets and sorrows of the past, to counteract all influences, all wishes and desires of the past and to bring us back into the present'.*

If there is one remedy that represents the Divinity found in each of the remedies, it is 'Star of Bethlehem'. This remedy is the remedy of comfort for pains and sorrows, according to Bach.† What better remedy for a constricted heart chakra? Traditionally always given for shock, trauma, and grief, this remedy seems to promote a release from the wounds that cause us the deepest of hurts. Physical traumas heal; but inasmuch as we are spirit in body, the wounds that cause us the deepest grief are those rooted within us emotionally – in other words, in our *heart*. These wounds have a symbiotic relationship to Star of Bethlehem that's divinely healing. On the spiritual level, the flower Star of Bethlehem presents a balanced image of six perfect petals of white, evoking the image of the aforementioned, spiritually significant six-pointed star, the perfectly counterbalanced triangles, the phrase 'as

*Chancellor, p. 111   †ibid., p. 179

above, so below' and the culmination of the colours in the spectrum. Often, I've heard this remedy referred to as the 'ultimate healer of all wounds' and 'the Divine Mother essence'. It truly is a remedy for a heart in distress.

On our evolutionary journey, it's paramount to keep in mind that the will to heal is the gateway to accessing our soul's purpose, lying within our spiritual heart. An additional key to this gateway is our ability to embrace and practise the act of forgiveness; forgiveness for ourselves and for others. To find that forgiveness within us requires surrendering the self-imposed guilt and shame attached to the contracted issues of the root, sacral and solar plexus chakras. Until we're able to give ourselves permission to take a different path from that of our family or tribe, to make our own choices and stand in our power within our external environment, we cannot extend forgiveness to others. When we have given ourselves these permissions, then we're better able to forgive others who have hurt us. As a bonus, we're burning the karmic debt necessary to move forward. In his book, A PATH WITH HEART, psychologist Jack Kornfield identifies forgiveness as:

> *One of the greatest gifts of the spiritual life. It enables us to be released from the sorrows of the past.... Forgiveness does not in any way justify or condone harmful actions.... Forgiveness is simply an act of the heart, and an acknowledgement that, no matter how strongly you may condemn and have suffered from the evil deeds of another, you will not put another human being out of your heart.*

Then, and only then, will we be able to ask the question, 'did I love enough, *unconditionally?*', and get a response that reverberates throughout our deepest levels of awareness.

*Kornfield, pp 284-5

NINETEEN

—

Speak Loudly, though your Knees Quake: the Fifth Chakra

Agrimony, Cerato, Larch, Chestnut Bud — Wisdom

'How does one become a butterfly?' she asked.
'You must want to fly so much that you are willing to
give up being a caterpillar.'
Trina Paulus, HOPE FOR THE FLOWERS

SOUND, BOTH spoken and heard, is the energetic element of the fifth centre, our throat. If we review the emotional patterns held within each chakra explored up to this point, we find that within each of them rest aspects of choice. In our first chakra, the root, we're faced with the issue of who will make choices for us? Will it be our tribe or ourselves who determine the direction our path takes? In the sacral and solar plexus, we find our choices affect our empowerment or disempowerment creatively; they shape our personal relationships, our self-esteem and our ability to function in our external environment. Finally, coming to this point on our mystical path, we find that the ramifications of the choices we've made in these centres culminate in our heart, affecting our spiritual health.

We now come to our fifth chakra, the throat centre. With this centre, we've arrived at a new frontier, the chakras related to our 'spiritual awakening'. And we're now embarking into the territory of what the ancients and spiritual teachings identify as the realm of ether or space. With this centre, we establish our relationship to the external earthly realm and the divine within us through 'sound'. The question before us is *what is the disposition of this relationship?*

In the previous chapters, we've learned that we must be faithful in our commitment to do our own emotional work in our lower centres. And, if we have done the work required for our spiritual progress and soul's evolution, we benefit from our labours in the throat chakra. This area of focus represents our ability to hear our intuitive wisdom and to speak it. In its highest expression, the fifth chakra is the place from which we put a voice to Our Truth by speaking out and speaking up.

The unfoldment of the throat chakra will lead the soul to a wider and deeper understanding of the eternal, unchanging truths of life. It is linked with the sense of hearing, both on the physical and spiritual plane, and with the vocal cords and the production of sound.'*

Still, emotionally and spiritually hearing our wisdom and then speaking it, is a formidable challenge when our first four chakras are in contracted states.

If we've not been able to shift the emotional patterns of the root, sacral, solar plexus and heart chakras into expansion, then this fifth centre will remain contracted in all aspects as well. Thus, *speaking our truth* can be fraught with difficulties, as it may be easier for us to speak our truth than to follow through with what we have said. An authentic journey requires fundamental commitment and action; not simply thinking and talking.

For some, when they actually have 'spoken up', they embed their authentic work in this very action. Back when I

*Hodgson, THE STARS AND THE CHAKRAS, p. 138

was in private practice as a Bach Practitioner and now in my current Evolutionary Astrology work, I've clients who find it very easy to speak up (or out), but doing the internal work required for authentic commitment is another matter. Red flags to making this commitment come in the form of words that 'ring hollow' or giving lip-service, such as verbalizing the current spiritual 'buzz' when, in actuality, the authentic process is missing.

Emotional contraction in the throat chakra inhibits us from asking for what we need, so we're unable to 'speak up'. But how can we 'speak up' if we've been disempowered in the other centres, unable to make choices for ourselves? This contraction prevents us from hearing our intuitive wisdom clearly. Unable to trust it, we're unable to verbalize it.

Being incapable of speaking our truth is only one manifestation of contraction in this centre. Again, sound is the operative characteristic of the throat chakra, and verbalization always carries with it an important responsibility. We choose words to express ourselves, and our words transmit powerful vibrations through the ethers. When the throat centre is contracted, our words can emit toxic vibrations to those around us and these vibrations reverberate back to us, creating yet more toxicity within.

In this centre, we find that the issue of choice remains within us and has to do with how we communicate our intent, desire, self-direction; our will. If we've done the work needed in our lower chakras, our throat centre will be ready to enter into a state of expansion. This enables us to hear our intuitive wisdom and speak our own high truth. In doing so, we verbalize the intentions of our soul's purpose, intentions that represent the balance of our feminine and masculine energies, which have been protected in our heart centre.

When we offer words with humble intent, with no expectations, we offer unconditional love in the name of universal connection and service. This doesn't mean everyone will accept what we have to say. The authenticity of unconditional love isn't determined by acceptance of our words. Individuation is critical for each of us, so it's important to keep in mind that on our journey we're not all reading from the same map; we're not meant to. The understanding of this principle was one that was very clear for Edward Bach and a concept repeatedly interwoven throughout his writing:

We must not expect others to do what we want, their ideas are the right ideas for them, and though their pathway may lead in a different direction from ours, the goal at the end of the journey is the same for us all. We do find that it is when we want others to 'fall in' with our wishes that we fall out with them.'*

From the physical perspective, a contracted throat chakra can manifest as problems in regions of the throat, teeth, mouth, hypothalamus and the vertebrae of the neck. Caroline Myss also identifies addictions as an indication of fifth-chakra difficulties.†

There are a number of remedies that can be considered when trying to expand a contracted fifth chakra, and each addresses distinctly different emotional issues. In Chapter Eight, we learned that Bach identified **Agrimony** and **Cerato** as soul type remedies. But these remedies also are indicated or useful when an individual manifests the negative emotions of either the temporary mood state or personality type of these remedies. In a constricted state, those manifesting the negative Agrimony mood or personality type live in intense internal turmoil by hiding their genuine feelings, uncomfortable with verbally expressing feelings of distress.

Back in Chapter Eight, we also saw how the negative

*Barnard, COLLECTED WRITINGS, p. 102   †Myss, ANATOMY, p. 98

state in Agrimony soul types can turn to addictions, particularly drugs and alcohol, as a means of self-medicating in order to manage their distress. The same can be applied to the negative mood state or personality type. As a healing tool, Agrimony helps to provide an individual with the feeling that they're in an emotional place of safety and therefore able to verbally express their needs or their distress successfully.

The issues of hearing intuitive wisdom, trusting it and expressing it, lie at the heart of the Cerato soul type, personality type and the mood state. The phrase, 'Know Thyself' was inscribed above the entrance to the Temple of Apollo at Delphi, in the sixth century BCE. In terms of the fifth chakra, we could expand this phrase to 'know thyself and speak it'. Such is the very essence of the high expression of Cerato. In the negative mood state or personality type, as is true with the soul type, the intuitive voice is heard only as a faint whisper. There's hesitancy in trusting this voice, and a further inability to verbalize it with confidence. As a result, time is spent doubting every choice made. This behaviour increasingly promotes an internal powerlessness and certainly promotes it externally, in the eyes of others.

Cerato as a remedy promotes the courage needed for effective external expression of inner knowing, of authentic judgment and intuition. The positive energy of the remedy shifts the internal perspective, thus amplifying the voice of intuition and inner knowing. In this space, the individual then holds the power of speaking their high truth.

The personality type and mood state of **Larch** was discussed in Chapter Seventeen. Having to do with issues of self-esteem (a third-chakra issue), we can also consider this remedy as a healing tool for a contracted throat chakra. If we don't possess self-esteem, this dysfunction will be verbalized through a smokescreen of toxic words. Such expression only serves to damage others and ourselves. In order to verbalize our desires and needs, self-esteem is essential, making Larch the remedy to call upon to assist us in this process.

In her book, THE STARS AND THE CHAKRAS, the astrology author Joan Hodgson states:

> *The unfoldment of the throat chakra will lead the soul to a wider and deeper understanding of the eternal unchanging truths of life.... As the throat centre becomes active, the soul begins to feel a longing to communicate — to sound its own individual note in the grand harmony of the universe ... [but with this] there can be a danger of mental pride and arrogance, barring the path to true spiritual union with the Divine which the soul seeks.* *

Here Hodgson cautions us not to let mental pride and arrogance interfere with our ability to make wise choices. When the fifth chakra is constricted, mental pride, arrogance, or a sense of entitlement prevent us from making choices with clear discernment or judgment. In its effort to teach us the importance of discernment in exercising our 'will', our soul provides us with repetitive opportunities through which we can test our progress. Some of the most visible illustrations of these 'soul opportunities' arise in toxic relationships or life situations based on unrealistic expectations. When finding ourselves in such circumstances, we can gauge our progress in learning the soulful skills of sound judgment and clear discernment by our ability to recognize these patterns and reject them.

Since the fifth chakra is about sound, if we continue to ignore our soul's messages through denial and resistance, we can hardly expect to speak with clarity. As a result, we have to rework this lesson until we 'get it'; and 'getting it' is imperative to discovering our soul's intended purpose for us.

*Hodgson, STARS AND CHAKRAS, p. 138

The remedy **Chestnut Bud** reflects both a mood state and a personality type. With Bach identifying his remedies in three categories – soul type, personality type and mood state – we're reminded that all twelve soul remedies can function as the other two, although he didn't consider the balance of the remedies as soul type remedies. To refresh here, a personality type remedy represents the chronic emotional state one's personality presents (which can vacillate between a positive and negative state), while the mood state is temporary. From this perspective, Bach believed that the personality type remedies and the mood state remedies were the ones to consider when addressing illness, reminding us that these remedies and the emotions they represent are very much about our reactions to our environment.

Chestnut Bud is the remedy Bach chose as the one to help us recognize our repetitive patterns of behaviour, the ones preventing us from developing clear discernment. By expanding our internal vision, Chestnut Bud has the ability to move us from a diminished state of detrimental repetitiveness into a more balanced state – and in this process, gives us an understanding of the consequences of our actions. Again, as with all the remedies, be they a soul type, mood state or personality type remedy, there must be a willingness to take part in our process. Spiritual teachings remind us that

> *The difficult part is for a soul to live, day by day, in a dark world absorbing the lessons which the outer life is intended to teach.... Humanity actually spends its time running away from itself, seeking dissipation and oblivion.... [Again, the] essential lesson ... that life has to teach humanity is to face itself.* *

As Hodgson implies, when we develop aspects of dis-

*White Eagle, THE LIGHT BRINGER, pp 82-4

cernment through these lessons, such as sound judgment, sensitivity, and insight into the choices we make, our fifth chakra expands and we move further along our soul path of purpose toward the acquisition of *Wisdom*.

TWENTY

It's Not in your Head: Lightbulb Moments, the Sixth Chakra

Cherry Plum and Aspen – Certainty

*'Use your imagination not to scare you to
death, but to inspire you to life'*

Anonymous

VISION, imagination, inspiration, and awareness of
our high truth are all channels our soul uses to inform us that we're making progress along our evolutionary path. The information we receive through these
routes comes in 'lightbulb moments' that give us glimpses
of this. Moreover, it's through the centre of the sixth chakra
that we 'receive divine light'. As a mystic and psychic, Edward Bach became especially sensitive and receptive to such
moments during the last two years of his life, particularly
with his discovery of the final nineteen remedies. But as early as 1931, when Bach wrote HEAL THYSELF, it can be seen
that he was aware of our potential sensitivity to the Divine
and our intuition, as he refers to such sensitivity as 'flashes
of knowledge and guidance [that are] given to us'.*

Making our way upwards through the upper triangle
of our chakra symbology, we find that this centre (located
above and between our physical eyes) is identified in eastern

*Barnard, COLLECTED WRITINGS, p. 147

philosophy as the 'third eye'. It is in this centre that we have potential access to an innate understanding of the unknowable. Successful transition into this 'place' however, requires that we have first transformed the emotional patterns of the first five chakras with authenticity; otherwise, it's certain that we'll continue to intellectualize our lightbulb moments and dismiss those that we can't explain through reductionist or mechanistic philosophy.

As we were reminded at the beginning of Chapter Eighteen, the ancient Egyptians believed that successful passage into the underworld was determined by an appraisal of an individual's heart centre against the feather of Maat, the goddess of truth, law, and universal order. Interestingly, we find that other spiritual traditions teach similar concepts although they are expressed differently:

> *Always remember that although words have their place, and are useful to open the door, you cannot advance into the Temple of Initiation on words alone! The passwords on the spiritual plane are not spoken words only. Passwords are sounded in the heart, and you cannot advance ... without sounding the password of the heart centre ... which is love.... You cannot have the power without being love.* *

Even if we've done our work in the lower chakras, transformation of the emotional patterns in the heart centre is particularly important to our progress, for living universal brotherhood/sisterhood is grounded in the heart. This said, we also need to remember that the power of words and sound, our words grounded in the throat chakra, do not guarantee us an automatic entrée into the place where we receive the 'flashes of knowledge and guidance' to which Bach refers. In order to 'receive' such knowledge, it's essential to

*White Eagle, THE LIGHT BRINGER, pp 82-4

remember that the success of our emotional excavations will be deliberated within the heart, whether we have lived past lives in ancient Egypt or are simply modern-day travellers. If we've been authentic in the emotional excavation of the lower chakras, and that of the throat, the positive energy of our worldly will in these centres facilitates our heart chakra to open and expand. As described earlier, in an ongoing flow, this expansion then rebounds throughout the other chakras in support of their own expansion. When our heart centre is open, it becomes a potent sacred space where fusion between the balanced emotional patterns of the other chakras can take place including a balanced sixth centre.

The vibrant emotional and spiritual energy of this chakra honours both our conscious and unconscious wisdom. Here, the language of its wisdom is one felt through the heart and then verbalized through our throat chakra. Furthermore, in this balanced state, we become open to lightbulb moments of *vision, imagination, and inspiration*, as we realize our high truth.

What's important to remember is that this sixth chakra is also connected to the power of the rational mind. When shut down, the mind emerges as the grasping, hungry ghost, greedy in its desire to dominate to our own detriment. In Bach's view, greed itself fostered a desire for power, manifesting in issues of control. He saw greed as the emotion denying the recognition that every soul has the right to freedom and individuality.* It's also interesting that he identified 'pride' as representing not only arrogance but also rigidity of the mind. Thus, we find that domination by our mind or intellect isn't really supportive of our journey toward soul awareness of purpose.

The intellectual mind doesn't understand the concept

*Barnard, COLLECTED WRITINGS, p. 132

of universal connection, even though this is the greatest lesson we need to learn as we make our way into the Aquarian Age. When our intellect dominates, our intuitive wisdom is cut off. Whether or not we're aware of it, we become prisoners of ourselves and dangerously stuck in our process. In this state, we cannot 'see'; we're blinded to our inner vision and knowing, making it impossible for us to hear the voice of our intuition.

When we engage in the emotional work necessary to expand the lower chakras, various forms of therapy discussed earlier can all be excellent tools – in addition to the various remedies suggested to this point. Each of these resources is a useful contributor to doing our inner work. Beyond the remedies and self-understanding through the soul's messages reflected in our astrological birth chart, other tools are available to us for expanding the upper chakras.

In a different category from the ones used in expanding the lower centres, one of the most powerful is the practice of contemplative prayer and/or meditation. Books, webinars, downloads and classes provide excellent resources for learning the various methods of meditation. Regardless of the paradigm one chooses, the object of meditative practice is to develop the skill of objective and silent introspection. Bach himself wrote on this subject, remarking:

> *The perfect method of learning [to obtain a faithful picture of ourselves] is by calm thought and meditation, and by bringing ourselves to such an atmosphere of peace that our Souls are able to speak to us through our conscience and intuition, and to guide us....* *

While the remedies are invaluable in assisting us in our quest, it's interesting that Bach is telling us, in so many words, that peaceful silence of contemplative prayer or meditation

*Barnard, COLLECTED WRITINGS, p. 147

is the key to being able to hear our intuitive guidance. This isn't a mental exercise, but one of the heart, and a message given to us by spiritual teachings as well:

> *When you are distracted by material things, keep very calm, keep very still.... Touch the silence and the power of the spirit will flow into you and disperse all your fears.... 'Nothing is so important as God.' There are many very clever people with great intellectual development, but despite all their knowledge, they are unable to penetrate the higher ethers or touch this profound spiritual silence; and indeed, until you have developed the required spiritual qualities, you will never penetrate these finer ethers.* *

Unfortunately, for some, their sacred shopping has derailed them and, as we've already seen, their desire to be 'spiritual' becomes so intense that they make their quest an intellectual one, rather than a spiritual one. It's safe to say that it's impossible to attain expansion of the sixth chakra and the ability to 'receive' through a frenzy of reading books, quoting biblical passages or proselytizing. Silence and authentic introspection are two of the major keys to the expansion of this chakra. We saw in the discussion concerning Bach's South Node karma, that service, in the name of unconditional love rather than ego, is yet another powerful key.

The emotional patterns of a contracted sixth chakra can manifest in a variety of dysfunctional and abusive behaviours such as rage, attempts to control others and dictatorial domination. Each of these has been discussed in relation to contraction of the other chakras. However, when the sixth centre is in a state of contraction, we can also become what psychologists refer to as delusional. Among the characteristics of this emotional state are illusions of grandeur, as described in various editions of the Diagnostic and Statistical

*White Eagle, THE LIGHT BRINGER, p. 39

Manual of Mental Disorders (DSM) which is a resource guide used by mental health professionals – especially in the United States. In other words, the individual can develop an inflated sense of worth, power, knowledge, or believe they have a special relationship with a deity or famous person.

When this happens, they can take on the mantle of a self-professed guru, which not only invites further derailment from their soul's intended path, but derails those whom they beguile as well. We build up access to our soul's purpose by doing our emotional work with the help of the remedies, our soul's map for this lifetime through our natal chart and introspective meditation. It's important to remember one more time that in working towards this access, with the help of these tools, the onus of work still lies with our active participation in our process. Solely relying on these resources to do our work will not reap the results we're after, any more than sitting in contemplative meditation as a phlegmatic observer will bring us enlightenment. I have met my share of false gurus. As Bach practitioner and now with my practice in Evolutionary Astrology, I have had clients who believe they're doing the necessary emotional work simply because they're taking remedies and/or have had chart readings from me. For anyone, success in their process requires working through the emotional patterns lodged in the chakras from a place of self-awareness and in an orderly fashion. This includes authentic mentors who have travelled the path a few steps before us. Make no mistake, they're no different from those of us who are 'learning the ropes'.

I tell my clients, 'the minute you hear grandiosity, experience abusive behaviour, language or any other suggestion that a mentor is more interested in you meeting their needs than the mentor supporting your growth, run the other way. Be especially alert to any needs for adoration on the part of your spiritual advisor or mentor.' This type of need, by 'another', isn't supportive of chakra expansion or health.

In addition to its links with our mental capacity, the sixth chakra is physically associated with our brain and central nervous system. When this centre is out of balance, we can experience neurological difficulties, seizures and/or learning disorders. From the spiritual perspective, these manifestations are giving us clues that a spiritual war is raging within us. This experience is not unusual during one of the major astrological 'life cycles' in a chart which happens around the age of 42.* On one hand the mind, fearful that it will lose its place of importance, is battling for its survival. On the other, our soul is trying to steer us into a place of awareness where we can access our highest truth and know what our soul's purpose is for this lifetime.

From a remedy perspective, these manifestations, emotional and physical, represent the classic struggle between soul and personality agendas. In Chapter Fifteen, the remedy **Cherry Plum** was introduced as a choice for a contracted first chakra. However, in the case of the sixth centre, when the mind is in its struggle for dominance over the soul, we can also consider this remedy. Cherry Plum was the remedy Bach described for the mind being overworked and unable to take 'strain'. An important consideration of Cherry Plum is its ability to promote internal resolution between mind and soul and thus foster a sense of peace.

Up to this point, the discussion regarding 'contracted emotional chakra patterns' has been intended to portray an image of centres that are 'closed' like the shutter in a camera just before the picture is snapped. Diverting from this

---

*Often denoting a 'spiritual crisis' (approximately at age 42), this event is known as the Uranus opposition when transitting-moving Uranus 'opposes' the position of natal Uranus in the chart.

concept, the sixth centre presents us with an inconsistency in our imagery. On one hand, when the sixth chakra expands as in the sense of demonstrating balanced emotional patterns, we have an opportunity to access vision, imagination and our high truth. Still, in this opportunity, we must remember this is also the centre that fosters our psychic abilities; and in this, there is an inherent danger in expansion, as in being too open.

Expanded in an unbalanced way, the sixth centre makes us susceptible and open to 'psychic attack' or 'psychic possession'. In this sense, although the sixth centre is expanded, it's actually out of balance and therefore in a state of contraction. If this is the case, we can experience a type of fear so irrational that we're afraid to verbalize it to others and lack the language to do so. Our intuition or 'sixth sense' is so skewed that the imagination, rather than being creative and balanced, reels out of control in unrealistic, emotionally destructive fantasies. In this state, our mind conjures up scenarios, events, and anticipations at a frenetic pace. This results in states of heightened anxiety and/or an intense fear of radical things happening around every corner. It's important to note that these emotions have no tangible basis. A patent and widespread example of this state was a way of being for most Americans in the days and months following September 11, 2001. More recently, an example is the flooding of social media by supporters of unfounded, deep-state conspiracies, creating a great deal of anxiety and suspicion around the validity of science amidst a global pandemic.

Barnard reminds us that when Bach discovered the final nineteen remedies, he left us with no evidence in his writings as to what specific circumstances initiated this last chapter of his work. The only clues we have are from Nora Weeks. As I pointed out in earlier chapters, she tells us that Bach experienced specific emotional states of distress just before discovering the remedy that balanced out each particular state of his distress. No doubt, Bach's psychic capabilities were finely tuned to a very high frequency at this point in his life (1935). Thus, it's reasonable to assume that he was susceptible to the implications of a sixth centre that had become too exposed to disquieting influences of a psychic nature. Being open to the etheric plane involves risk for anyone, and this was no less true for Bach. Therefore, we can also reasonably assume that this was his experience leading to his discovery of the remedy **Aspen**.

Bach described the negative Aspen state as experiencing

> '*an unknown mental fear that comes over you like a cloud, bringing fear, terror, anxiety and even panic without the least reason. These fears are often accompanied with trembling and sweating from the object of fear of something unknown.*' *Conversely, he maintained that the positive attributes of the Aspen remedy promote 'fearlessness because of the knowledge that the universal power of love stands behind all. Once we come to that realization, we are beyond pain and suffering, beyond care or worry or fear; we are beyond everything except the joy of life, the joy of death, and the joy of our immortality.... We can walk [our] path through any danger, through any difficulty unafraid.*'*

As we strive to obtain a 'faithful picture of ourselves', as Bach called it, we must consciously be aware that balance is of the utmost importance in this particular centre. And, when we achieve this balance, spiritual teachings tell us there are marvellous rewards. Open to vision, inspiration, imagination, our high truth, and a 'different way of knowing', we're reminded once again that all great work is done quietly and with **certainty**.

*Chancellor, p. 43

When the soul has acquired all the lessons necessary, when it has attained a degree of completeness, it puts forth a more complete presentation of itself. Then you are able to see and recognize a master, an adept, an initiate. *

*White Eagle, TREASURES OF THE MASTER WITHIN, pp. 113-14

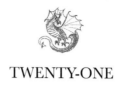

TWENTY-ONE

—

Illumination: the Seventh Chakra

Sweet Chestnut, Star of Bethlehem — *Faith*

'Come to the edge', he said. They said, 'we are afraid'.
'Come to edge', he said. They came.
He pushed them... and they flew'
Guillaume Apollinaire

IN THE NATIVE American tradition, young men, and sometimes women (depending on the tribe) undergo a spiritual ritual known as a 'vision quest'. When successful, this ritual of initiation brings the initiate to a place of temporal balance and spiritual adulthood. Though the specifics vary, typically the process includes rituals of purification followed by an intense journey of solitary introspection into the etheric realms. Aided by their spirit guide or animal, this 'journey' provides 'a focus and sense of purpose, personal strength, and power.' In the shamanic tradition, briefly discussed in Chapter Sixteen, vision quests are also undertaken in cases of individual problematic circumstances or issues affecting the entire tribe.

The ritual of a sacred journey into the etheric realms is not exclusive to the Native Americans but is part of every culture and tradition under various labels. For example, in the Christian tradition, one could identify Christ's forty days and forty nights in the desert as his personal 'vision quest'. Within this framework, the upward journey we make through the emotional patterns of our chakras can be considered our personal vision quest in search of our soul's evolutionary purpose for this incarnation. The culmination of this journey is the apex of the upper triangle in our chakra symbology. Identified as the seventh chakra centre of *illumination*, it's located at the crown of our head. When this centre is in a state of expansion, we're open to the integration of unconditional surrender to the wisdom of, and faith in, the Divine in every cell within our physical body and every vibration of our etheric bodies.

This is illumination, and it's the Golden Apple sought by the spiritual seeker. At the very heart is our ultimate connection to all that's Divine within and without us. Thus so 'enlightened', we come to recognize our high truth. *Now* we have the opportunity to embrace this and, in doing so, radiate light to others. However, in our attempts to reach this point of completion, we still can face difficulties.

For some, impatience develops with the pace of their progress. As a result, they're tempted to evade remnants of the emotional work needed. This temptation results in something like a short circuit, wherein through inappropriate practices the person forces the *kundalini*, the divine fire (or cosmic fire, as it is sometimes called), to rise prematurely up through the other chakras. In eastern philosophy, the symbol of this cosmic fire or energy is a coiled serpent lying dormant within the root chakra, at the base of the spinal column. Spiritual teachings inform us that the *kundalini* power is centred in the heart and that through gentle meditation, proper spiritual awakening calling for the arousal of this latent energy can be achieved in an orderly ascension up through the chakras, beginning with the root. When we become impatient and attempt to bypass the orderly work needed for this process, serious physical problems can result.

According to Carolyn Myss, such imbalances include those within the central nervous system, the skeletal system, and muscular system of our body. These are red flags for a seventh chakra whose state is precarious. Imbalances can manifest in energetic disorders, mystical depression, sensitivities to the environment and chronic exhaustion that isn't linked to a physical disorder*

Typically, such disorders are subject to an array of biologically-based diagnoses by those trained in the western medical tradition. Unfortunately, in these situations, the problem arises in that recommended treatments rarely solve the problem. It isn't that the methods of western medicine are substandard, but simply that until a few years ago, most western-trained physicians weren't educated in treating such imbalances from a mind/body/spiritual perspective, something eastern philosophy and medicine have considered imperative for thousands of years. Once again, on this issue of how to treat illness and disease, we find that Bach was a visionary in his approach to illness. A saying of his that's well-known within Bach circles is, 'treat the person, not the disease'. Here he was directly referring to our emotions as the foundation of illness.†

So we find, despite some progress on our journey, that we still may have some remaining demons and dragons to slay. Therefore, acquiring the Golden Apple of Union with the Divine doesn't appear to be imminent. Typically, these dragons are the ones that continue to lurk in the comfy lairs of our lower centres. Because we haven't yet banished them, we still have work to do.

*Myss, ANATOMY, p. 101

†It should be noted that Bach made exceptions to this approach in the case of circumstances such as catastrophic accidents.

Imbalances in the seventh centre can create disillusionment and disconnection, throwing us into what St John of the Cross called the Dark Night of the Soul. Quite simply, we believe that we're in a state of spiritual abandonment. The key here is that we still haven't emotionally grasped the concept of faith in unconditional surrender to the Divine. The classic description of the negative **Sweet Chestnut** state is 'dark night of the soul'. Those in the throes of this state experience unbearable anguish and the perception of assured annihilation. This is a most desperate emotional state for anyone. For those in this state, the abyss before them can create emotional, physical, or spiritual paralysis, and it's not uncommon for someone to experience all three simultaneously, because this chakra centre is either totally contracted or intensely out of balance.

Bach identified the Sweet Chestnut remedy as the one for 'that terrible, that appalling mental despair when it seems the very soul itself is suffering destruction. [It is] the hopeless despair of those who feel they have reached the limit of their endurance.' Clearly, Bach must have experienced this state to describe it so. He goes on to say that the positive action of this remedy enables those, despite their anguish, to reach out to the Divine. To this end he said, '... the cry for help is heard and it is the moment when miracles are done.'*

If we find ourselves surrounded by the darkness of our abyss, Sweet Chestnut is the remedy that creates the light we need in order to for us to see through this darkness. Barnard refers to the Sweet Chestnut remedy as the one that is able to 'pull consciousness up from the darkness of [the] underworld.'

In addition to Sweet Chestnut, it's useful to remind

*Chancellor, p. 186

ourselves of the remedy Bach referred to as the 'comforter of pains and sorrows', **Star of Bethlehem**. While the specifics of this remedy have been covered in Chapter Eighteen, it's interesting to contemplate the image of the flower, Star of Bethlehem, and all the flowers that Bach chose for healing, within the concept of spiritual teachings:

> *There is nothing haphazard in creation, all is perfection – perfect rhythm, perfect form, exactness in every detail.... Take a tiny star-like flower, and place it under a microscope, and you will see it as a jewel, you will see all the colours of the rainbow reflected in its petals, and if you are attuned to the harmonies of the spheres of light, you will hear them sounding from the beauty of that little flower.... Look for beauty in your everyday life. Do not take things for granted. Look for the exquisite beauty in flowers, in the sunlight, in the dewdrop.*†

So, in order to realize illumination rather than illusion, our seventh centre must be in brilliant and harmonious expansion with our other chakras. For this to happen, it's imperative that we have trust and unconditional faith that there is a Divine Plan, a Soul Purpose for each of us, expressly orchestrated to inspire transformation that balances us physically, emotionally, and most importantly, spiritually.

*White Eagle, SPIRITUAL UNFOLDMENT II, p. 100

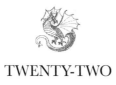

TWENTY-TWO

—

Keeping on Keeping on: Joining Heaven and Earth

The spiritual journey is one of continually falling on your face, getting up, brushing yourself off, looking sheepishly at God, and taking another step.

Aurobindo

THE CENTRAL theme for humanity in the Aquarian age is internal harmony with our Divine Self and the external harmony of universal connection. While our soul holds this wisdom, some of us – most of us – have disconnected from this wisdom in our frenzy to speed toward and through the wonders of technology. As a mystic and healer, Edward Bach knew that nature is symbiotic with our soul's agenda. This is something the ancients intuitively knew long before the age of technology. They *knew* that all life-energy is connected. And they *knew* that it's the Divinity of nature and the heavens that enfolds and balances us on all levels in our quest for connection to our soul's plan for us.

Long before Copernicus and Galileo were considered heretics by lesser men, the ancients were intuitively aware that our body and spirit were connected to the pulsating rhythm of the night sky. As far back as the third millennium BC, their primal observation of the heavens planted seeds of modern astronomy and astrology. This underlines the fact that Evolutionary Astrology is esoteric astrology at its very core. As such, this specialization of western astrology is nothing less than a reflection of spiritual law laid down by our soul as a blueprint for our evolutionary journey this lifetime.

In our process, the flower remedies of Edward Bach, our astrological birth chart and an understanding of the importance of the energy in our chakra centres move us toward the surrender and faith necessary for our soul's growth. In the most subtle of ways, these tools help us step out of a space that imprisons us emotionally. They provide us with the prospect of emotional safety by fostering personal introspection and connection to our perceptions and behaviour. In essence, they say to us, 'this is difficult work, but you are safe in doing it'.

Bach maintained that our soul holds the innate wisdom of each of us. However, when we spiral into the lower emotional expressions of our natal Moon, become stuck in the emotional energy of its South Node, or when our chakras and their emotional patterns contract, this wisdom becomes clouded. It is as if a curtain of fog drops over this wisdom and we are unable to 'see' clearly. Dr Bach's remedies help to lift this fog, shifting our perception to a more realistic state of clarity so that we may take the 'next right step'.

It's through this very action that they assist us in reclaiming our place on our mystical path, providing us opportunity and giving us a vision of the intimate relationship we have with the spiritual realm. They help us tap into our reality so that we understand who we are in our quest to discover and manifest our soul's purpose, as laid out in our birth chart. For Bach, the understanding of our spiritual reality was his *high truth*.

Within the realms of cosmic law, there's the concept of soul age, similar to the concept of our physical age in the mundane world. As we travel the cycle of birth, death and rebirth, we have many opportunities to learn valuable soul lessons and as we stumble, get up, dust ourselves off, move on, and sometimes succeed along the way, our soul ages in wisdom. Edward Bach was not only a mystic and healer. He was a great soul, an old soul.

Bach's gift to us was one of selflessness. Such a gift is an important quality that is necessary in all of us if we're to achieve the divine mandate of universal connection in brother–sisterhood. While those who worked with him admit he was not always an easy person to be with, his capacity for compassion towards all other human beings was paramount.

As we learned in Chapter Eleven concerning the Nodal Axis of Bach's natal Moon, we're reminded that it's safe to imagine this triggered his intuitive consciousness of having a specific job to do in this incarnation. With the added awareness that time was fleeting, it's realistic to assume this was what drove him in his states of impatience and intensity. Although he paid a high price physically, his insatiable passion to find a means of helping others heal their minds and bodies through nature was his mission. For him, finding our soul path and discovering our purpose and connection to the Divine were the reasons for being.

We'll never know the intimate details of Bach's personal 'flashes of knowledge and guidance' that led him to his discoveries. Regardless of this, the foundation of his work and his words are clearly anchored in spirit. He repeatedly urges us to manifest all that we *are* in spirit. Over and above his work as a physician, this was his reason for being. His own wisdom informs us that our healing and soul growth depend upon the balance of our emotional energy. For Bach, the life force or positive energy of nature held the keys to healing, understanding of our soul's purpose and growth. The 'flash of knowledge' we get as the keys turn, this is the divine alchemy of universal connection, brotherhood and unity between all peoples.

For these things, our gratitude to Edward Bach is immeasurable.

> *The gaining of our freedom, the winning our individuality and independence, will in most cases call for much courage and faith. But in the darkest hours, and when success seems well-nigh impossible, let us ever remember that God's children should never be afraid, that our souls only give us such tasks as we are capable of accomplishing, and that with our own courage and faith in the Divinity within us victory must come to all who continue to strive.*
>
> Edward Bach, M.B., B.S., M.R.C.S., L.R.C.P., D.P.H.

AFTERWORD

SHORTLY BEFORE his death, at the early age of 50 in 1936, Bach wrote several letters to friends, colleagues and business associates that seem to imply he was 'tidying up things' in preparation for his transition. Certainly, since he was a physician, it's not unreasonable to assume he was well aware of his physical status. But in the following letters , one gets the sense that Bach was in a place far outside the density of the physical realm:

> *I am expecting a call to a work more congenial than of this very difficult world.... The Work I have put before you is Great Work, it God's Work, and heaven only knows why I should be called away at this moment to continue to fight for suffering humanity.* *

And this, written only one month to the day before his passing.

October 26, 1936

Dear Folk,

It would be wonderful to form a little Brotherhood without rank or office, none greater and none less than the other, who devoted themselves to the following principles:

> *1. That there has been disclosed unto us a System of Healing such as has not been known within the memory of men; when, with the simplicity of the Herbal Remedies, we can set forth with the certainty, the absolute certainty, of their power to conquer disease.*

> *2. That we never criticise nor condemn the thoughts, the*

*ORIGINAL WRITINGS, ed. Howard and Ramsell, p. 173

opinions, the ideas of others; ever remembering that all humanity are God's children, each striving in his own way to find the Glory of his Father. That we set out on the one hand, as knights of old, to destroy the dragon of fear, knowing that we may never have one discouraging word, but that we can bring hope, aye and most of all, certainty to those who suffer.

3. That we never get carried away by praise or success that we meet in our Mission, knowing that we are but the messengers of the Great Power.

4. That as more and more we gain the confidence of those around, we proclaim to them we believe that we are divine agents sent to succour them in their need.

5. That as people become well, that the Herbs of the field which are healing them, are the gift of Nature which is the Gift of God; thus bring them back to a belief in the love, the mercy, and the tender compassion and the almighty power of the most high.

Edward Bach*

*Barnard, COLLECTED WRITINGS, p. 170

AUTHOR NOTE

WHEN I WAS an active Bach practitioner, two of the questions I would often hear from my clients and those who attend my workshops were, if Bach was such a great healer, what did he die from and why did he die so young? From a physical standpoint Bach's health was always an issue and as discussed in this book, his death certificate notes cardiac failure and sarcoma. However, from a spiritual perspective, mystics and visionaries often 'sense' that the time for their earthly work is drawing to a close and do not fear their transition. Through these writings directed to his closest companions and associates, that we can see this was no less true of Edward Bach.

THE THIRTY-EIGHT BACH FLOWER REMEDIES

Alphabetical List

Agrimony*
Aspen
Beech
Centaury*
Cerato*
Cherry Plum
Chestnut Bud
Chicory*
Clematis*
Crab Apple
Elm
Gentian*
Gorse
Heather
Holly
Impatiens*
Larch
Mimulus*

Mustard
Oak
Olive
Pine
Red Chestnut
Rock Rose*
Rock Water
Scleranthus*
Star of Bethlehem
Sweet Chestnut
Vervain*
Vine
Walnut
Water Violet*
White Chestnut
Wild Oat
Wild Rose
Willow

The asterisk indicates the Twelve Healers and Soul Types

ASTROLOGICAL BIRTH SIGNS

Western System. There are slight date variations from year to year and depending on location

Aries (March 21 - April 19)
Taurus (April 20 - May 20)
Gemini (May 21 - June 20)
Cancer (June 21 - July 22)
Leo (July 23 - August 22)
Virgo (August 23 - September 22)
Libra (September 23 - October 22)
Scorpio (October 23 - November 21)
Sagittarius (November 22 - December 21)
Capricorn (December 22 - January 19)
Aquarius (January 20 – February 17)
Pisces (February 18 – March 20)

SELECTED FURTHER READING
EDWARD BACH & MIND, BODY, SPIRIT HEALING

Dr Bach's own writings are to be found assembled by Julian Barnard in his COLLECTED WRITINGS, below, and in the edition of ORIGINAL WRITINGS, edited by Judy Howard and John Ramsell, listed below under their own names.

Bach, Edward. COLLECTED WRITINGS OF EDWARD BACH. Ed. Julian Barnard. London: Ashgrove Publishing, 1987.

Ballantine, Rudolph. RADICAL HEALING: INTEGRATING THE WORLD'S GREAT THERAPEUTIC TRADITIONS TO CREATE A NEW TRANSFORMATIVE MEDICINE. New York: Harmony, 1999.

Barnard, Julian. BACH FLOWER REMEDIES: FORM AND FUNCTION. Hereford: Flower Remedy Programme, 2002.

Dr Philip M. Chancellor's HANDBOOK OF THE BACH FLOWER REMEDIES, Keats Publishing, New Canaan, Ct. 1971

Dossey, Barbara. florence nightingale: MYSTIC, VISIONARY, HEALER. New York, Lippincott, Williams & Wilkins, 1999.

Gerber, Richard. VIBRATIONAL MEDICINE FOR THE TWENTY-FIRST CENTURY: THE COMPLETE GUIDE TO ENERGY HEALING AND SPIRITUAL TRANSFORMATION. New York: Eagle Book, Harper Collins, 2000.

Hasnas, Rachelle. THE ESSENCE OF BACH FLOWERS: TRADITIONAL AND TRANSPERSONAL USE AND PRACTICE. Freedom, Ca.: Crossing Press, 1999.

Hay, Louise. YOU CAN HEAL YOUR LIFE. Santa Monica, Ca.: Hay House, 1984.

Hodgson, Joan. ASTROLOGY: THE SACRED SCIENCE. Liss,

Hampshire: The White Eagle Publishing Trust, 1978.

—, THE STARS AND THE CHAKRAS. Liss, Hampshire: The White Eagle Publishing Trust, 1990.

Howard, Judy, and John Ramsell. THE ORIGINAL WRITINGS OF EDWARD BACH. Essex: C. W. Daniel Co., Ltd., 1990.

Kornfield, Jack. A PATH WITH HEART: A GUIDE THROUGH THE PERILS AND PROMISES OF SPIRITUAL LIFE. New York: Bantam, 1993.

Myss, Caroline. ANATOMY OF SPIRIT. New York: Harmony Books, 1996.

—, WHY PEOPLE DON'T HEAL AND HOW THEY CAN. New York: Harmony Books, 1997.

Rinpoche, Sogyal. THE TIBETAN BOOK OF LIVING AND DYING. Patrick Gaffney and Andrew Harvey, Eds. San Francisco: HarperCollins, 1993.

Teasdale, Wayne. THE MYSTIC HEART. Novato, Ca.: New World Liby., 2001.

Weeks, Nora. THE MEDICAL DISCOVERIES OF EDWARD BACH, PHYSICIAN: WHAT THE FLOWERS DO FOR THE HUMAN BODY. Essex: C. W. Daniel Co., Ltd. , 1973.

White Eagle. THE LIGHT BRINGER: THE RAY OF JOHN AND THE AGE OF INTUITION. Liss, Hampshire: White Eagle Publishing Trust, 2001.

—, THE PATH OF THE SOUL: THE GREAT INITIATIONS. Liss, Hampshire: White Eagle Publishing Trust, 1997.

—, TREASURES OF THE MASTER WITHIN. Liss, Hampshire: White Eagle Publishing Trust, 2002.

—, WHITE EAGLE ON THE GREAT SPIRIT. Liss, Hampshire,:White Eagle Publishing Trust, 2003

ASTROLOGY

Arroyo, Stephen. ASTROLOGY, KARMA AND TRANSFORMATION. CRCS Publications, 2nd ed. 1992

Clow, Barbara Hand. UNDERSTANDING YOUR KEY LIFE PASSAGES: LIQUID LIGHT OF SEX. Bear & Co. Publishing 1991

Cunningham, Donna. ASTROLOGY AND VIBRATIONAL HEALING. Cassandra Press 1988

—, HEALING PLUTO PROBLEMS. Red Wheel/Wisner 1986

Forrest, Steven (http://www.forrestastrology.com). THE INNER SKY, Seven Paws Press 1988 (previously published by Bantam Books, Inc., 1984)

—, THE CHANGING SKY. Seven Paws Press 2008. ACS Publications, second edition 1998, second edition (previously published by Bantam Books, Inc., 1986

—, YESTERDAY'S SKY, Seven Paws Press 2008

—, THE BOOK OF THE MOON. Seven Paws Press 2010

—, the elemenst series. Seven Paws Press:

  —, THE BOOK OF FIRE. 2019

  —, THE BOOK OF EARTH. 2019

  —, THE BOOK OF AIR. 2020

  —, THE BOOK OF WATER. 2020

Hand, Robert. HOROSCOPE SYMBOLS. Whitford Press 1981

Sasportas, Howard, THE TWELVE HOUSES. Flare Publications (London School of Astrology) 1985

CITATIONS IN TEXT NOT
FOUND IN 'FURTHER READING'

Bell, Rudolph M. HOLY ANOREXIA. Chicago: Univ. Chicago Press, 1997

Cameron, Julia. THE ARTIST'S WAY. New York: Tarcher, Putnam, 1992.

HARPER'S ENCYCLOPEDIA OF MYSTICAL AND PARANORMAL EXPERIENCE. 1991.

Ingerman, Sandra. 'Medicine for the Earth, Medicine for People", in *Alternative Therapies in Medicine and Health* 9:6 (2003) 77-84.

Mack, Gaye. 'Exploring Implications of Treating Eating Disorders with Vibrational Medicine as an Integrative Therapy.' 1999, DePaul University., Chicago, Illinois.

White Eagle. *Stella Polaris*, 1952, pp 18–19, 184.

– , SPIRITUAL UNFOLDMENT II. Liss, Hampshire: White Eagle Publishing Trust, 2002

ACKNOWLEDGMENTS

IN THE EXPLORATION of the Moon's zodiacal sign in Chapter Ten the subject of teachers and mentors who show up for us on our evolutionary path was introduced. Sometimes in the moment we don't recognize them as such only to discover years later, how important they were to our self-discovery of soul purpose.

And then there are those whom we do recognize. In both categories my list is long, but I have no doubt looking back there are more realizations to come and in future, those I've not yet met. For now however, particularly regarding this book, I have a few mentors who deserve special mention.

During my Bach years I had the privilege of several wonderful and especially gifted teachers in Dr Bach's work. My American teacher, Elisabeth Wiley who taught my Practitioner Levels I & II through the Dr Edward Bach Foundation, was an amazing woman. For many years on, I had a continued correspondence with her, appreciating her economy of words in getting her wisdom of experience and insights across. In 1996 Lynn MacWhinnie, Bach author in her own right and international teacher for the Bach Centre, was sent to Chicago to teach myself and others what at the time was the final Practitioner Level course. Although so many years ago, we continue to have a friendship across the vastness of the Atlantic. Twenty-five years on, I can still see her drawing Chinese characters on a whiteboard to make her point about compassion in our class. Years later in an effort to expand my knowledge, I spent a wonderful week out in California attending a Practitioner Intensive led by Patricia Kaminsky and Richard Katz at their 27-acre Terra Flora gardens and wildlife centre. As founders of the North American Flower Essences repertoire, known as FES, they've always been respectful of Dr Bach's work in their own work and dedication, which added another layer to my knowledge.

Back in 1988 when THE INNER SKY by Evolutionary Astrologer, Steven Forrest, was released, I devoured it, never dreaming that years later I'd enter a face-to-face apprenticeship with him. In the interim twenty-one years, I focused on my Bach work, floating in and out of my fascination with astrology which I'd had since days as an undergraduate. This included a brief time spent in study with the London Faculty of Astrological Studies. At the time, their style of teaching wasn't a fit for me and so I abandoned that avenue.

As I noted in Chapter One, events for me took their own course after nearly twenty years working with the Bach remedies. With the universe in the driver's seat, I was thrown back to astrology but this time, head first into my apprenticeship with Steven which continues to this day. To say he's been one of my most important teachers and mentors on my own journey is an understatement.

I mentioned in Chapter Ten about those who are on the same path as we, but walking just a few steps ahead. And yet in this, he never forgets to reach back and pull us along through his face-to-face teaching, writings and generosity of time to answer some really stupid questions, sprinkled with his unique brand of humour.

While we know there are no coincidences or accidents around those who cross our path in this incarnation, my debt of gratitude for my teachers in the Bach work and especially to Steven Forrest for his mentorship of my work in

Evolutionary Astrology, is deep.

Although I'm no longer an active Bach practitioner, my practice in Evolutionary Astrology is global. Should you wish a reading with me, please check out: www.gayemack. com or contact me directly (gayemack@gayemack.com). I would love to work with you in finding out not only 'who' you are, but also 'why' you are in the self-discovery of your evolutionary purpose.

And as always, appreciative of Colum Hayward and Polair Publishing for once again bringing the work of Edward Bach to the forefront and, this time, with a new look through the lens of Evolutionary Astrology.

GFM, August 2021

INDEX